Healthy Eating and Pollution Protection for Kids

What Every Parent Should Know About
Safe-guarding the Health of Their Children
in the 21st Century

David Reavely

Healthy Eating
and
Pollution Protection
for Kids

What Every Parent Should Know About
Safe-guarding the Health of Their Children
in the 21st Century

David Reavely

BOOKS

Winchester, UK
Washington, USA

First published by O-Books, 2011
O-Books is an imprint of John Hunt Publishing Ltd., Laurel House, Station Approach,
Alresford, Hants, SO24 9JH, UK
office1@o-books.net
www.o-books.com

For distributor details and how to order please visit the 'Ordering' section on our website.

ISBN: 978 1 84694 621 9

A CIP catalogue record for this book is available from the British Library.

Design: Lee Nash

Printed in the UK by CPI Antony Rowe
Printed in the USA by Offset Paperback Mfrs, Inc

We operate a distinctive and ethical publishing philosophy in all
areas of our business, from our global network of authors to
production and worldwide distribution.

CONTENTS

I would like to dedicate this book to world renowned naturopath and author Jan de Vries, who has always supported me in my efforts to spread the word about the importance of healthy eating.

Since we live in a world that presents us with many health challenges including exposure to junk foods and pollution, this is not an easy task. Not only has Jan supported me, he is at the forefront of natural medicine, and continues to carry on the legacy of that other iconic advocate of nature cure, world famous herbalist and naturopath Alfred Vogel.

Acknowledgements

Looking back, it occurs to me that over the years many adults and children have influenced me in terms of providing the motivation to write a book on healthy eating and pollution protection for children. This partly came about due to my early experiences and interaction with pupils and fellow teachers in the 1980s and 1990s, many of whom motivated me to try and get the healthy eating message out there to as many people as possible.

I feel particularly grateful to Broomhill Bank School in the south of England, as my contribution towards their healthy eating policies was always encouraged and appreciated.

Special thanks also to my partner Jenny, who has always encouraged me in my writing endeavors and to whom I have always turned to for advice and support.

Foreword

"Yet again, this is another good book from Dave. His books are irresistible because he speaks from the standpoint of practical knowledge, and all the information embodied within this book makes it a truly valuable addition to every household!

I admire Dave for his continued efforts to bring the latest research into his books.

His advice for every parent will provide the tools to help children stay healthy, and is an easy read. It is my fervent hope that the reader will apply the good advice given in this invaluable book."

Jan de Vries Author and natural health guru appearing on television programs including Richard and Judy's 'This Morning' and 'Open House with Gloria Hunniford'

Introduction

The fact that the title of this book attracted your attention suggests that you are serious about giving your children the best start in life. If you're interested in feeding your children with healthy food and protecting them from pollution in order to promote their good health, as well as increase their resistance to the majority of chronic diseases that plague the Western world then join the club.

You are definitely one of a growing body of adults who are becoming seriously worried about the effects of junk food and environmental toxins upon our precious children. If, like me, you are determined to do something about it, then I sincerely hope that you are successful in your quest. I am also hopeful that this book will help to provide you with at least some of the tools that every parent needs in order to get their kids eating healthily.

One thing that I would like to acknowledge right from the beginning is that getting your precious one's to ditch the 'junk' and start to eat healthily is not easy. Please believe me when I say I'm speaking from experience here! As a father of two children, I spent many an hour chopping up vegetables and attempting to prepare healthy meals; and let me tell you that the recipients were not always appreciative of my efforts.

What's more, this was during a time when healthy eating wasn't quite so well accepted as it is nowadays. Jamie Oliver – where were you when I needed you? I can also tell you that I made quite a few mistakes along the way.

Of course in one respect this harsh training ground was a good thing, because the precious knowledge that I gained during this period served me well when writing this book. Hopefully it will help you to avoid making the same mistakes.

Finally, let me explain that this book came about as a result of an absolute determination on my part to get the healthy eating message across to as many children, parents and teachers as possible. I believe that knowledge can empower people. It can help them to make informed choices; and when you make the right choices, you can influence your life!

David Reavely
Cert Ed. Bed (Hon), DN Med, MBANT

1

Perils of the Western Diet

I've talked to a lot of parents over the years who genuinely believe that they feed their children healthily. Usually the conversation goes something like this:

Me: "Would you say that your kids eat healthily then?"

Parent: "Oh yes, they eat their vegetables and are quite fond of fruit; well, mostly bananas actually."

Me: "Sounds good. What about the likes of bread and pasta?"

Parent: "Yes, they eat lots of bread; mostly sandwiches, that sort of thing. My oldest boy practically lives on pasta. Still, they say it's good for giving you lots of energy don't they?"

Me: "What kind of bread and pasta is it? Is it whole meal or the white variety?"

Parent: "Oh, it's usually white bread and white pasta. We've tried getting them to eat whole meal but they can't stand the stuff!"

Me: "Ok, what about protein foods?"

Parent: "Yes, they get plenty of protein. My youngest girl Michelle, she eats loads of cheese, bacon, and ham. Oh, and she likes her beef-burgers, but not too many; maybe three times a week."

Me: "They don't eat nuts, seeds, peas or beans then?"

Parent: "I'm afraid not. Well, apart from salted peanuts, but I suppose they're not too healthy are they?"

Me: "True, salty foods are definitely not recommended I'm afraid. What about sugary foods?"

Parent: "Well, I have to admit that they do like their sweets."

Me: "What, chocolate, that kind of thing?"

Parent: "Oh yes, they must get through loads of the stuff. I've tried getting them to cut back, but they just get all irritable and grumpy. I gave in trying after a while."

Me: "What about snacks?"

Parent: "Yes, they do need snacks. I'm trying to get them to eat more fruit. The trouble is they'll only eat a piece of fruit if they can have a packet of crisps afterwards."

Me: "How about drinks?"

Parent: "Well, I've been trying to get them to drink more water recently; but that's definitely an uphill battle. They're so used to drinking their fizzy drinks, which I know are not good. Still, I suppose it all balances out in the end."

Me: "Would you say they are quite healthy?"

Parent: "Well, to be honest, they're not as good as they used to be. I've noticed that they've had a lot more coughs and colds recently. My youngest boy has had lots of time off school of late. He seems prone to getting tonsillitis. With the others it's more mood swings, and spotty skin; but I've just put that down to their age really."

When you read about this kind of scenario you may think that it represents an extreme case. Sadly, in my experience, it is becoming increasingly common. What is so disturbing is that the parents who feed their precious children with this kind of 'foodless food' are unaware of the damage they are inflicting upon them.

Think of heart disease, cancer, obesity, diabetes and a whole host of other chronic conditions and you begin to get the message.

So what can we do to change things for the better? Well the first step is to try and get away from all of the confusion. For example, when it comes to healthy eating, one of the common statements I hear from people is: "We hear that this food is good for us on the TV one day, only to read in some newspaper the following week that this same food is bad for us! What are we supposed to believe?" This is a fair comment.

A good example would be chocolate. Is it good for us? Or is it bad for us? Some studies seem to support the idea that chocolate is good for us because it contains antioxidants that help to protect our cells from damage. Well, when we study the composition of the cocoa bean from which chocolate is derived, this does appear to be true. It is indeed packed with healthy antioxidants which are good for us. But let us now delve a little deeper.

In order to make delicious chocolate you have to add other key flavor-enhancing ingredients; these being sugar to give chocolate its sweet taste, fat to make the chocolate set; and if it's milk chocolate, milk or milk solids to give it that rich creamy taste. I'm sure you can see where I'm going with this? That's right, these other ingredients change what is essentially quite a healthy but fairly unpalatable food, into a delicious unhealthy food because it contains sugar (usually lots of the white refined variety), full-cream milk, which is high in saturated fat, and worst of all, the type of vegetable fats often added to chocolate are the hydrogenated variety, which are really bad for us.

Now, if we take a long hard look at a lot of other processed foods, we'll find the same kind of scenario emerging. Take the case of white flour, for instance. This starts off as whole wheat grains which naturally contain all the goodness of the wheat. These grains are crushed by steel rollers and then separated into their component parts; namely, the wheat germ (which contains lots of vitamins and minerals), the white starchy endosperm, and the bran (the part of the wheat that gives us valuable fiber). Guess which part is used to make white flour? Yes, that's right, the white starchy endosperm. This is the least nutritious part of the wheat and merely provides us with energy from the starch which is converted by the body into sugar. Therefore, anything made from this kind of flour is devoid of whole food goodness. In fact, white bread which is made from refined flour, not only lacks any real nourishment, it also contains chemical additives, so it is one of the unhealthiest foods one can eat.

These two examples help to explain why so much confusion exists on the subject of nutrition these days. What it often ultimately boils down to is this: foods are usually better for us when they are least interfered with. When we analyze the types of refined foods that constitute the so-called Western diet, it is not hard to conclude that the human body was never meant to consume them in the first place.

In order to understand this fully we only need to remember one key fact: we are part of the animal kingdom; and this being the case, it beggars the question: what other animal living in its natural habitat lives on junk food?

What We Can Learn From Some of Our Furry Friends

When it comes to understanding the importance of living on natural foods in contrast to unnatural refined foods, one has only to consider the example of the black bear, an animal that is native to Canada. Black bears are omnivorous and their diet consists of about 75 percent vegetable matter, 15 percent carrion, and 10 percent insects and small mammals. Their love for honey is well known. They also have a liking for ripe corn in the autumn.

As you might imagine, providing that this magnificent animal has access to such natural foods, it remains healthy and disease-free. What's more, with the exception of grizzly bears and man, it has few enemies. In some parts of North America, they are hunted.

However, another threat comes from tourists who feed the bears with junk food. When this happens the bears develop a taste for these unhealthy foods and are tempted to invade campsites and tourist centers in search of more.

Unfortunately, like us humans, the consumption of too much of this kind of food can result in the bears becoming sick. This doesn't just apply to bears of course; it also applies to other wildlife such as deer and wild cats.

So what is the message here? Well, the parallels are obvious when we focus on the fact that we humans are a part of the animal kingdom, and like our fellow creatures we were meant to live on natural foods. There is plenty of evidence to suggest that if we do live on a natural diet, then we are far less likely to suffer from all of the major chronic diseases.

Still need convincing? Well perhaps the following true story may reinforce this point.

The Story of the People of Hunza

Hunza is a state situated in the extreme northernmost point of India. For many years the people who lived in this remote and then inaccessible region were renowned for their impressive longevity and good health. The late Sir Robert McCarrison, who was a pioneer of nutritional research, lived amongst them for a number of years. During this time he observed that their diet consisted of unrefined wheat, barley, maize, vegetables and an abundance of apricots. These were dried in the sun and formed a large part of their diet.

In studying the health of the Hunza people, Sir Robert observed that their diet was very pure, and although they lived a very frugal existence, they suffered from virtually none of the diseases that are so prevalent in modern society. Cancer, diabetes, strokes and heart disease were rare.

What eventually happened to these people should be a lesson to us all. With the advent of civilization came better access to this remote and mountainous region. This led to imports of processed foods such as white sugar, white flour and alcohol. Unfortunately this corrupted their pure and natural diet, and for the first time in their history they began to suffer from the type of chronic diseases that appear to be accepted by our modern society.

If ever there was a lesson from the past that we should heed, then surely this is it!

In fact the message could not be more emphatic:

We were meant to live on natural foods, designed by nature to provide us with all the elements we need to sustain good health!

We were not designed to live on unnatural processed foods such as those made with white flour, refined sugars, unhealthy fats, high in salt and laced with additives.

If we ignore these natural laws, then we become significantly more vulnerable to chronic disease.

What is interesting is that the same principles that influenced the longevity and promotion of good health amongst the Hunza people, also appear to be having the same positive effects on other races that live close to nature. For example, the natives of

Vilcacamba in southern Ecuador, the Abkhasia of the old Soviet Union and the Okinawans of Japan. There are some differences in terms of the types of foods they eat; for example soy beans feature in the Okinawan's diet. However, the common denominator seems to be that they all eat plenty of fruits and vegetables as well as other natural unprocessed foods such as whole grains, pulses and a small amount of animal protein.

Needless to say, chemical additives and unhealthy fats are not a feature of their diet. Nor are they exposed to the same levels of pollution compared to many of us around the world. The end result is that they live longer more active lives and are less likely to suffer from the killer diseases so prevalent in Western society.

So, as parents, what is the lesson here? In essence, the frightening situation exists whereby millions of parents around the world are unwittingly inflicting damage upon their children as a result of wrong-feeding. The vast majority would be appalled if they knew the overall impact of their actions; for like you and I, they are caring and loving parents who just want the best for their children. However, despite the difficulties, it doesn't have to be this way. We can bring up our children to appreciate the link between the correct choice of food and health. We can also teach them to respect nature, to gain an understanding of where our food comes from and to acknowledge our place in the ecosphere.

2

So Just What is a Healthy Diet?

Are you trying to get the children in your family to eat healthy food? Do you find it all a bit daunting? Are you worried about making the right choices? If this sounds like you, then this chapter may help to make your life a lot easier.

As I stated in Chapter 1, when it comes to eating healthily, the most important thing to remember is to select foods that have been least interfered with and to avoid or minimize the one's that have been processed the most. Foods such as white flour and white sugar definitely come into this category. When the time comes for you to plan your food shopping list, it's a good idea to apply the natural versus unnatural principle in order to help you select the healthiest foods for your kids. In order to help you I have devised a table of unhealthy foods and their healthy counterparts. You can use this as a quick reference guide.

OMIT/MINIMIZE	BETTER OPTION
White wheat flour and all products made from it such as white pasta, spaghetti, macaroni, noodles, etc	Whole wheat flour and its products such as whole wheat bread and cookies, brown pasta, spaghetti
White rice, white rice noodles	Whole grain rice, brown rice noodles, brown rice flour (for cooking)

Other grains that have been refined such as corn, buckwheat	Their whole grain equivalents, e.g. whole grain corn, buckwheat noodles made from whole grain buckwheat.
White and light brown sugar (sucrose), golden treacle, high fructose corn syrup, any other refined sugars	Honey, molasses, black treacle, very dark sugar in small amounts, date syrup
Dried fruits preserved with sulfur dioxide or any other chemical preservatives such as potassium sorbate	Dried fruits (preferably organic) free from preservatives
Refined breakfast cereals made with refined grains such as cornflakes, sugary puffed white rice	Breakfast cereals made from whole grains such as whole grain corn, whole wheat puffs, whole grain rice, whole oats, porridge, muesli
Processed cheese containing chemical emulsifiers and preservatives	Unprocessed cheese made without artificial additives
Fizzy drinks containing sugars and/or artificial sweeteners and/or caffeine	Natural fruit juices made from 100% pressed juices; e.g. apple, pineapple, orange. Dilute 50:50 with pure water.
Foods fried in polyunsaturated oils, such as sunflower, safflower, rapeseed, etc	Foods briefly fried in extra virgin olive oil, coconut oil, or 'steam fried'

Sweetened canned fruits (these usually contain sugar syrup – refined sugar)	Canned fruits sweetened in their own juice or sweetened with apple juice, grape juice
Coffee and tea	Rooibosch tea (this is caffeine free), herb teas, coffee substitutes (e.g. chicory). Sweeten with a little honey or date syrup, if desired
Spirit vinegar, malt vinegar, acetic acid and foods pickled in them	Cider vinegar, balsamic, wine vinegar (cider vinegar is generally regarded by nutritional practitioners as the healthiest), pickled foods using these vinegars
Heavily spiced foods	Mildly spiced foods and those flavored with herbs
Heavily salted foods; table salt	Low salt foods. Foods lightly salted with sea-salt or Himalayan salt
Rich and fatty meats, processed meats (e.g. corned beef), luncheon meat, commercially produced sausages, burgers, ham. These are likely to contain preservatives such as sodium nitrite	Unprocessed meats (preferably organic) such as lean chicken, turkey, home-made sausages, burgers

Smoked or cured fish such as smoked haddock, salmon	Fresh fish, canned fish without chemical additives (e.g. wild salmon)
Chocolate	Chocolate alternatives, such as carob; a small amount of quality raw chocolate made from healthier fats and higher in cocoa solids
Savory snacks made with refined carbohydrates and high in salt, unhealthy fats and additives such as monosodium glutamate	Savory snacks made with whole grains, non-hydrogenated fats and other natural ingredients; lower in salt and additive-free. For example, naturally flavoured corn chips.
Roasted salted nuts; with additives such as monosodium glutamate and artificial flavorings.	Unsalted nuts and seeds. These contain healthy fats which are otherwise destroyed in the roasting process. Good choices include walnuts, pecans, hulled hemp seeds, pumpkin seeds, etc.*
Cereal and fruit bars packed with sugar and chemical additives	Cereal and fruit bars that have no added sugar and are made with only natural ingredients, such as dates, raisins, coconut, molasses, oats, quinoa

Canned and packet soups containing artificial additives, refined wheat flour, sugar	Fresh carton soups made with natural ingredients, without added sugar, artificial flavorings or refined wheat flour

* Warning
Not suitable for very young children due to risk of choking; also not suitable for children with nut or seed allergies.

The Importance of Fruits and Vegetables

The thing to remember is that every time you feed your child fresh fruit and vegetables, especially in their raw state, you are supplying them with an abundance of vitamins, minerals, anitioxidants, amino acids, enzymes and a whole variety of essential nutrients that work together, synergistically, to bring about good health. Synergistically meaning they work even better together as the whole is greater than the sum of their parts.

This is why, ideally, the bulk of your child's diet should consist of fruits and vegetables, with at least 50% in their raw state. It's worth remembering that raw foods contain enzymes and other natural compounds that are destroyed by heat. Therefore, although some cooked vegetables can be nutritious when cooked with minimal heat, generally speaking, they are not quite as nutritious as raw foods.

Daily Eating Plan for Children – Key Points

- Include at least one salad a day as part of a meal or on its own

- Eat at least 3-4 pieces of fruit per day. If your child doesn't like many types of fruit, see if they will drink a freshly-made smoothie

- Include a variety of multicolored foods such as red bell peppers, squashes and carrots. These are rich in health-promoting and protective phytochemicals.

- Include foods like broccoli, watercress, sweet potatoes and sprouted seeds (eg. alfalfa, sunflower, aduki bean or mung bean sprouts) as these are rich in antioxidants which are health-promoting and protective against cancer.

- When cooking foods try to steam as much as possible; or use the steam-fry method.

- Feed your child with as many whole foods as possible and minimize their consumption of processed and refined foods.

- Buy organic foods whenever possible. If using commercially-grown fruits and vegetables, peel skins or throw away outer leaves and wash the vegetables thoroughly.

- Include some fermented foods such as live yoghurt, miso and sauerkraut.

- Give your child a good multi vitamin and mineral supplement on a daily basis (see 'Useful Information' at the end of this book).

- Use only pure filtered water or spring water for drinking purposes.

- Include whole grains such as brown rice, quinoa, oats and whole wheat or rye, rather than refined grains, such as white flour.

- If meat is included in the diet, select naturally reared chemical-free, organic, and free-range meat and choose mostly white meats such as chicken. Avoid cured and processed meats such as corned beef, ham and bacon. These foods contain chemical additives and are high in salt, and the additives may be carcinogenic.

- Try to include some oily fish such as wild salmon, sardines and mackerel twice or three times per week. These can be made more child-friendly as home-made fish cakes and fish pie.

3

Keeping Them Sweet!

Give Me the Sweet Stuff

Give me the sweet stuff, I want to be high!
Cos baby sugar's my ticket to fly!
It makes me feel good; it makes me feel free,
It gives me a quick fix of energy!
So give me my chocolate and all things so sweet,
Let me be hyper to all those I meet!
They say what goes up, has to come down,
So when I eat sugar, whether white or the brown,
I'm gonnah feel flat, like I'd been on some drug,
I'm gonnah slow down like the proverbial slug!
One minute I'm buzzing, and dance to the beat,
The next I feel empty, and life ain't so sweet!

David Reavely 2006

Let me begin this chapter by making an important statement:

We were not designed to eat sugar in its isolated form.

Generally speaking, sugar is a form of carbohydrate that has been isolated from the plant which it came from. Take sucrose, for instance. This is the chemical name for white and brown sugar. Now there's a processed food if ever there was one. This form of sugar is either derived from the plant sugar-cane, or sugar beet.

This is what happens when sugar-cane is processed:

- The sugar-cane is harvested and transported to a factory to be processed.

- The first part of the extraction process produces a very dark sticky substance called molasses. As well as being rich in natural sugars such as fructose and sucrose, it is also rich in minerals such as potassium and iron. It is also high in B vitamins.

- The next part of the extraction process produces black treacle, which is still quite high in nutrients, but tastes sweeter as it is higher in sugar.

- The black treacle is further processed to produce golden syrup. As you might imagine, this substance doesn't have any real nutritional value since most of the nutrients have been processed out of it. What is left is very sweet, sticky syrup which is mainly composed of sucrose.

- The final part of the extraction process produces a pure white crystalline substance, otherwise known as white sugar. This is the stuff we sprinkle on our breakfast cereal, add to our tea or coffee, or use to sweeten our bakery products.

- It is also the principle sweetener in confectionary products, the most popular being chocolate. It gives us a quick burst of a 'sugar high', but is virtually devoid of any nutrients.

As you can see from the foregoing description, as with most processed foods, we start with a natural substance that has some nutritional value. This food is then processed, and as a result, the end product loses most if not all of its nutritional value. What we then end up with is an edible substance that is completely changed from its original natural state.

More often than not it has been changed from a healthy food to a harmful one. In effect, white sugar has had around 90 percent of its vitamins and minerals removed.

Of course, we all consume sugar in other forms too. For instance, sugars such as dextrose (corn sugar), corn syrup, fructose (fruit sugar) and glucose are sometimes referred to as hidden sugars because they are added to many everyday foods. These everyday foods could include ketchup, pickles, mayonnaise, pasta sauce, tinned and packaged soups, breakfast cereals, curry sauces and peanut butter. Even bakery products such as bread often have some form of sugar added to the dough.

No wonder children get hooked on the stuff from an early age.

Why Are Our Children Eating More Junk Foods?

SUSTAIN, a pressure group that campaigns to protect children from advertisements that promote unhealthy foods, studied television advertising during children's viewing times. Their findings revealed that up to a staggering 99 percent of food and drink products advertised contained high levels of sugar, fat and salt. The biggest food category was sweets, cakes, chocolate (candy) bars and biscuits.

If we take a look around any supermarket, we are confronted with dozens of products that are designed to catch the eye of our vulnerable children. Most of the major manufacturers make big profits from selling such products, and you won't be surprised to know that they aren't too concerned about feeding children with healthy foods.

Sugar's Affect on the Health of Our Children

When we eat a chocolate bar, or some other food that is high in concentrated sugar; the sugar level in the blood rises rapidly. This creates a response from the pancreas, which secretes the hormone insulin. The insulin then enters the bloodstream where it comes into contact with insulin-sensitive tissues, such as muscle and fat cells. These tissues then absorb the sugar (glucose), resulting in a fall of blood glucose levels. This is desirable because it maintains a blood glucose level of around 90mg per decileter. In other words, insulin reduces the level of blood sugar by directing it into the cells. This is important, because if the sugar was allowed to remain in the blood it would jeopardize our health.

The problem arises when an individual becomes insulin resistant. When this happens, normal levels of insulin do not have the same effect, resulting in blood glucose levels remaining higher than they should be. To compensate for this the pancreas is stimulated to produce more insulin. Eventually, if this situation persists, it can lead to Type 2 diabetes.

In 1929, Dr. Frederick Banting, the scientist who discovered insulin, stated:

"In the US the incidence of diabetes has increased proportionately with the per capita consumption of sugar."

It's a frightening thought but the incidence of diabetes has tripled since 1958. It's now quite common to know of someone who is diabetic, yet around a hundred years ago it was rarer than a flawless George Bush speech.

Over the last few decades Type 2 diabetes, which is controlled with oral medication, has increased markedly. It is also becoming more common in children. Bearing in mind the increasing trend for children to consume 'junk' food, this is hardly surprising.

Obesity and Other Illnesses Associated with Sugar Consumption

Another major problem associated with sugar consumption is that of childhood obesity. Again this is a growing area of concern and the Government in the UK and in the USA have launched initiatives in order to try and address this problem. No doubt the fact that children exercise less has had an influence when it comes to regulating their weight; however, it is known that sugar is one of the biggest culprits since it is very high in calories.

Put simply, most obese kids eat foods that provide energy in excess of the body's requirements. The body's reaction is to convert the excess sugar into fat. The same thing happens with all refined carbohydrates such as white flour (and anything made with it such as white spaghetti and pasta) and white rice, since such foods, being absent in fiber, are quickly converted to sugar by the body. Is it any wonder then that in our junk food orientated society, obesity is at an all-time high?

Of course we know that over-weight children often have a tough time. Not only do they often lack self-esteem, but this is compounded by the fact that that they frequently become the victims of bullying from their peers. But let us not lose sight of the fact that childhood obesity brings with it the increased risk of such chronic conditions as heart disease, increased risk of cancer and strokes, later in life.

Although it sounds somewhat simplistic, childhood obesity can be overcome if children are fed a natural diet, comprising of foods known to be less calorie dense, such as vegetables, sprouted seeds, lean meats, fish, pulses and some fruits. These foods are an ideal antidote to the high fat, sugar and refined carbohydrates that feature in the so-called Western diet. Combine this with more physical activity, and you will have a winning formula.

Children have also had to pay another high price for their spiraling sugar consumption – their teeth.

Most folk are aware that good old sucrose damages teeth; but did you know that honey decays teeth faster? No wonder that the honey bear is the only animal found in nature that has a problem with tooth decay.

If you thought that diabetes, tooth decay and obesity were the only conditions that are caused by sugar consumption; you are in for a big surprise.

Take a look at the following list of sugar-related health problems:

- Sugar can suppress the immune system.

- Sugar can upset the body's mineral balance.

- Sugar can contribute towards hyperactivity, anxiety, depression, learning difficulties anxiety and behavioral problems in children.

- Sugar can lead to hypoglycemia (low-blood sugar) in children.

- Sugar can lead to chromium and copper deficiency.

- Sugar interferes with absorption of calcium and magnesium.

- Sugar can increase the risk of coronary heart disease.

- Sugar can reduce high density cholesterol (the helpful type of cholesterol).

- Sugar can promote the elevation of harmful cholesterol.

- Sugar can cause mood swings due to widely fluctuating blood sugar levels.

- Sugar can raise adrenaline (stress) levels in children.

A Word About High Fructose Corn Syrup

This is corn syrup that has been processed using enzymes to convert its glucose into fructose (fruit sugar). The next stage involves mixing it with corn syrup; hence the name, high fructose corn syrup. Sometimes dubbed Devil's candy, this sticky syrup is used in a wide range of products, including fizzy drinks, ice-cream, cookies, cereal bars and candies. Food manufacturers love it because it is cheap and has the property of retaining moisture, which extends shelf-life.

It will often be listed on a products list of ingredients as 'glucose-fructose syrup', 'high fructose corn syrup' and even 'HFCS'.

Some nutritionists are of the opinion that this sweetener tricks the brain into thinking you need more food. In addition, it is linked with triggering fat cells around vital organs such as the liver and heart. It seems that the glucose component is responsible for artificially raising appetite. Dr Carel Le Roux, a consultant in metabolic medicine at Imperial College London, explains it this way:

"When we eat sugar, our body releases insulin and other gut hormones which tell the brain that we have had enough to eat. High insulin and gut hormone levels are one of the factors that dampen the appetite. But fructose doesn't trigger as much of an insulin or gut hormone response as regular sugar, so the brain won't get the message that you are full."

Apart from tricking us into eating more than we should, high fructose corn syrup has been associated with health problems such as raising blood fats known as triglycerides, which are linked with increasing the risk of heart disease. What's more, some experts are coming to the conclusion that the syrup is linked with an alarming rise in diabetes.

The answer to this problem is to check food ingredients carefully and avoid high fructose corn syrup wherever possible.

Nature Knows Best

Now, having read the foregoing you might well ask the question: "Is all sugar bad for us?" Thankfully this isn't the case, because natural unrefined sugars are found in many of our everyday natural foods, such as fruits and vegetables. Carrots contain natural sugars, which is why they taste sweet. The same is true of vegetables such as parsnips, beetroot, sweet potatoes and onions. In fact, even quite bland tasting vegetables like celery and cucumber contain some sugars.

Of course, fruits are higher in sugars (mostly fructose), which is why they are more sweet. Since we derive energy from eating these foods, as well as important nutrients such as vitamins and minerals, they are an important part of a healthy diet.

Now here is another key point: Our primitive ancestors never had a problem with the over- consumption of sugar because the sugar they consumed was packaged in fiber. So when they ate fresh fruit, the fiber ensured that the sugars were released slowly, this resulted in a steady rise in blood sugar levels that gradually subsided as the body used up the sugar for energy. Not so with the likes of refined sugars such as sucrose (white and brown sugar). This quickly floods the blood with sugar stimulating the production of insulin from the pancreas. This results in an almost instant energy high.

However, there is a price to pay, since it is followed by a slump in energy levels as the blood sugar level dips when the insulin kicks in. This is why sugar-dependant children experience such wide mood swings, since such fluctuations in blood-sugar levels affect the brain, which depends upon a constant blood sugar supply to function properly.

No wonder children have been observed to concentrate better at school when fed healthy foods instead of junk foods.

Satisfying Your Child's Energy Demands

When it comes to satisfying your child's energy demands it is important to provide the correct type of carbohydrates. Bearing this in mind, try to encourage your child to eat the following foods:

- Choose whole grains such as 100% whole wheat pasta, bread, whole grain rice, rye bread, quinoa, oats and millet. They contain complex carbohydrates that are slowly converted to sugar and therefore provide long-term energy that doesn't stress the pancreas.

- Introduce more fresh fruit, such as apples, pears, mangoes, kiwi, pineapple and cherries. The sugars from these foods are released more slowly since they contain fiber. Berries such as blueberries and strawberries have minimal impact on raising blood sugar levels; so they make a great snack food in between meals.

- Use dried fruits such as dates, sultanas, raisins and apricots, but only in moderation as they are high in concentrated fruit sugar, and whilst this is better than consuming refined sugars, it can still elevate the blood-sugar level too quickly. Also, dried fruits are sticky and tend to stick to the teeth, raising incidence of tooth decay; so it is a good idea for children to rinse their mouth with water immediately after eating dried fruit.

- Fruit juices are a good source of vitamin C and antioxidants, particularly when they are made from pressed juice and not just made up from concentrates. There are lots of different flavors and combinations to choose from these days. I was surprised to see watermelon and kiwi juice in my local supermarket recently. All juices should be diluted with pure water on a 50:50 basis. Drinking through a straw helps to protect teeth from the fruit acids in the juice. You will need to limit their consumption though, as even diluted, they deliver a higher amount of fructose compared to eating a whole fruit, such as an apple.

- Encourage your child to develop a taste for fresh crunchy vegetables such as carrot sticks, celery and raw cauliflower. If you can introduce these foods at a young age then you'll be helping your child to develop a taste for natural foods that will stay with them for life. With older children it's still worth persevering because a liking for the natural flavors in foods can be developed when highly salted, flavored and processed foods are significantly reduced in the diet. The big advantage with eating these high fiber foods is that they do not adversely interfere with blood sugar levels and they really help to satisfy appetite.

- Pulses such as chick-peas, lentils and haricot beans are great for regulating blood sugar levels, as they contain complex carbohydrates (starch) and protein which the body has to convert into sugar for energy. A healthy version of baked beans sweetened with concentrated apple juice instead of sugar (sucrose) is a good alternative to the commercial varieties (available from many supermarkets and health food shops).

- Nuts and seeds are a good snack food, providing there are no allergy problems, since they are a wonderful source of long-term energy, and a good alternative to sugary foods. They are also a great source of essential fatty acids, so lacking in children's diets these days. Essential fatty acids are used by the brain, and are also an important building block for the central nervous system and nerve pathways.

You can also introduce children to nut and seed butters such as almond, pumpkin and sunflower. These can be used in the same way as peanut butter; e.g. spread on whole wheat toast or rye crisp-bread.

Warning
Since young children can choke on nuts and seeds it is wise to grind them in a grinder in order to avoid this danger. You can also used hulled hempseeds which are rich in protein and healthy fats – great sprinkled onto breakfast cereal or yoghurt.

What About Fruit Consumption?
Children should include a variety of fruits in their everyday diet – apples, pears, cherries, pineapples, guava, mango, grapes, melons, strawberries, blackberries, raspberries, blueberries, and so many other 'exotic' fruits. Children love smoothies, smoothie ice lollies, and fruit sticks (cubes of melon, pineapple and straw-berries threaded onto a wooden skewer kebab stick). Not only are they a delicious way to get into good habits, fruits are also a valuable source of antioxidants, phytochemicals, vitamins, minerals, natural sugars and fiber. The bulk of the diet should consist of vegetables with a smaller amount of fruits.

Fruit and Dental Care
Fruits have different levels of acidity. Some are very acidic, like lemons and oranges. When teeth are exposed to the fruit acids in fruits, the enamel becomes temporarily softened. The enamel will then become hard again after about 30 minutes. Therefore, children should be discouraged from brushing their teeth before this time has elapsed, since to do so will result in increased tooth decay as enamel is worn away. This is why fruit drinks and smoothies should be drunk through a straw, which reduces the amount of tooth exposure to the juice. Whenever possible, I would suggest that you encourage your child to drink some

water immediately after eating fruit or drinking smoothies and juices in order to rinse the teeth and minimize the effect of the acid and sugars.

This is especially so with acidic citrus fruits and dried fruits which are sticky as well as sweet, and will tend to stick to the surface of teeth. So, rinsing with water after they are eaten and then brushing after 30 minutes is a good way of preserving your child's teeth while enjoying the benefits of the vitamins, minerals and antioxidants they contain.

4

Adding In-salt to Injury

First the good news; we can get all of the sodium we need to stay healthy if we eat natural foods in addition to some food products that are seasoned with a little salt. The bad news is that most of us get too much sodium in the form of sodium chloride (common salt) which is added to everyday foods such as bread, biscuits, cheese, packaged foods, condiments, snacks and canned foods (e.g. baked beans).

Unfortunately children are exposed to lots of salt in almost everything they eat. The end result is that their taste buds get used to highly salted foods. When this happens they lose the ability to appreciate the more subtle flavors of natural foods such as fruit, raw vegetables and unsalted nuts and seeds. What's more, such high salt consumption increases the risk of high blood pressure, stroke and heart disease in their adult lives.

How Much Salt Should Our Children Consume?

A trace of salt is needed for the electrolyte balance and so a limited amount of salt in our diet won't harm us since the excretion of any excess is handled by the kidneys. This is important because there needs to be a balance in the body between sodium and potassium, since these minerals work closely together. In health, we should have around 92 grams of sodium in the body; around half of this amount is found in the fluids that surround our cells.

Now here is the interesting bit: in a healthy person the fluid that surrounds the cells is higher in sodium compared to potassium; however, the fluid inside our cells contains mostly potassium. This situation is carefully controlled by mechanisms in the cell membrane, sometimes referred to by nutritional practitioners as the 'sodium pump'.

When we consume too much salt this mechanism can malfunction and this results in excess sodium flooding into the cellular fluid and the cell losing its potassium. This culminates in damage to the cell's internal structure, including the mitochondria, which provide energy for the cell. The end result is a lowering of overall energy in the body and dehydration.

So, if your child often complains of feeling tired and listless, then it isn't necessarily just sugar and refined carbohydrates that are to blame; excess sodium can also figure in the equation.

Currently we consume on average, at least two and a half times what we need. Government public health campaigns have been trying to reduce average salt consumption for adults from more than 9g a day to 6g or less. Most authorities agree that it should be less for children, and the recommendation is as follows:

- Babies from 0-6 months = less than 1g per day

- 7-12 months = 1g per day

- 1-3 years = 2g per day

- 4-6 years = 3g per day

- 7-10 years = 5g per day.

These are maximum levels of salt and I would advise parents to aim for less. By ensuring that the diet is high in fruits and vegetables, the level of potassium will be kept high in relation to sodium, which is a desirable situation.

Thinking of the principle of a natural diet versus junk in relation to choosing what is good for our health, you won't be surprised to know that in nature, most fruits, vegetables, nuts, seeds, grains and other natural foods, are higher in potassium compared to sodium.

In other words, this is yet another example of nature knowing best. Therefore, it stands to reason that if we feed our children with mostly natural foods and make a point of purchasing foods that are low in salt, then we are helping their bodies to maintain a natural sodium and potassium balance.

Food Labels

Looking at food labels can be confusing. Basically you should be looking for the level of sodium in the contents. Generally speaking 0.5g per 100g is considered high, below 0.5g is moderate and 0.1g is low. Many manufacturers are now listing the amount of salt in an average portion, thus making it a lot easier to work out the levels.

In 2003, the Scientific Advisory Committee on Nutrition (SACN) concluded that since 1994 the evidence for a link between salt intake and blood pressure had increased. If you want to find out more I would suggest that you download the full **SACN** report on salt and health.

Tips for Cutting Down on Your Child's Salt Consumption

- Choose foods which are mostly low-salt foods – like chicken breast rather than ham, wild Alaska salmon rather than smoked salmon, sardines rather than smoked herrings.

- Choose snacks with a naturally low salt content such as rice cakes and rye crackers or home made popped corn to satisfy their need for a 'crunchy snack' instead of a packet of crisps or a processed salty snack.

- Encourage your child to eat unsalted nuts and seeds instead of the salted variety.

- Encourage a taste for natural foods such as fruit, raw vegetables (eg. carrot sticks, cucumber, cherry tomatoes, red bell pepper, raw cauliflower and mange tout)

- Don't put salt on the table to discourage the habit of adding salt to meals

- Don't add salt as a habit while cooking, unless the recipe specifically requires it. Many health food shops sell low-salt alternatives such as A.Vogel's very low-salt condiment that is based largely on potassium salts, which is far healthier.

- Try to develop your child's taste for herbs and mild spices to flavor foods, rather than always relying on salt

- Opt for fresh or frozen vegetables instead of canned, which have added salty brine.

- Rinse canned foods packaged in brine such as tuna to reduce their salt content.

- Avoid processed popular breakfast cereals which are surprisingly high in salt. Choose puffed whole grain rice with nothing added, or have a go at making your own muesli using ingredients such as oat, wheat, rice and buckwheat flakes; add your child's favorite fruit, either as dried fruit or fresh fruit, nuts and seeds.

5

A Fat Lot of Good

If you want to reduce the likelihood of your kids succumbing to arthritis, heart disease, hardening of the arteries, low energy, eczema, poor concentration, problems associated with the immune system, cancer and hyperactivity, then feed them fat.

Fat is good for them. Before you come to the conclusion that I have well and truly lost the plot, I hasten to point out that I'm talking here about good fats, otherwise known as essential fats because they cannot be made by the body.

For this reason such fats have to come from the foods we eat. Of course we all know that some fats, eaten to excess, can be very harmful to our health. I'm referring here to saturated fats, which are found in the likes of milk, butter, cheese and meats. We also have refined fats called trans-fats which are found in processed food products as mass-produced biscuits, cakes, chocolate, most margarine, pies and pasties, fried foods like donuts and fast food fries, and many other packaged foods.

Basically, most children brought up on a typical Western diet eat too many saturated fats and not enough of the healthy fats. Saturated fats are implicated as a major causative factor in the development of heart disease, thrombosis, hardening of the arteries, high levels of bad cholesterol, obesity and probably a whole host of other degenerative illnesses.

Types of Fat – Dispelling the Confusion
Put simply, all fats are made from fatty acids. These are basically the building blocks of fats, and some fats are vital in the body. Fat is not just found as a spare tire around the abdomen. It is a vital component in the body, in the brain and around the nerve

sheath protecting the spinal cord, for example.

Fats are made from a line of carbon atoms in the form of a chain, a bit like a caterpillar. Now imagine each carbon atom having side branches (like the legs of the caterpillar) to which a hydrogen atom is attached.

Now here is the scientific bit: each of these fats is classified according to how many of the side branches are taken up with hydrogen atoms. So, if all the branches are filled, then this type of fat is saturated.

As the name suggests, monounsaturated fat is not completely saturated and has just one space for one hydrogen atom. When it comes to polyunsaturated fats, I think you'll now be getting the picture, as indeed the name suggests, polyunsaturated fats are not 'saturated' with hydrogen atoms, since there are a number of sites around each fat molecule where hydrogen atoms could be attached, but are not.

Now just to complicate things slightly, there is another type of fat known as a trans-fat. Trans-fats are formed when polyunsaturated fats (e.g. safflower or sunflower oil), which should be good for you in their natural unprocessed state, are exposed to hydrogen gas.

As you can imagine, this saturates the fats with hydrogen atoms, which can be useful in food processing because it results in making the fats more solid at room temperature. For this reason, food manufacturers love the stuff because it is cheap to make, it doesn't deteriorate quickly (as polyunsaturated fats do) and it can be used in many everyday products such as chocolate, pastries and margarines.

The problem with this type of fat is that it has been shown to raise so-called bad cholesterol (known as LDL cholesterol) in addition to interfering with normal cell function. Fortunately, people like you and me are becoming more aware of the dangers associated with consuming trans-fats, and this consumer power has led to them being used less and less in products such as margarines, processed foods. Nevertheless, it is still worth reading the food labels carefully to ensure that the product you intend to buy is free from saturated or trans-fat.

What You Need to Know About the Main Types of Fat

From a health point of view it is perfectly acceptable to have all three types of fat in your child's diet as well as your own. The important factor, however, is getting the balance right. Basically, saturated fats get a bad press these days due to their link with raising cholesterol levels, which in itself is associated with a higher risk of cardiovascular disease. However, in my opinion, a small amount of saturated fat, say from butter or yoghurt made from whole milk, is not going to present a problem in small amounts; that is, providing the rest of the diet is good.

In terms of monounsaturated fat (for example from olive oil and avocados), the general consensus is that they are favorable in a healthy balanced diet since this type of fat is associated with lowering bad cholesterol (e.g. linked with blocking the arteries) and raising good cholesterol (e.g. in the brain). This would explain why the Mediterranean diet, which is high in olive oil, is believed to promote the health of the heart and blood vessels.

Moreover, unlike polyunsaturated oils such as sunflower oil, which can deteriorate during cooking at high heat, olive oil is believed to be healthier for cooking purposes (e.g. in stir-frying or tomato sauces).

This is because monounsaturated fats, due to their partial saturation with hydrogen atoms, are much more stable when heated and are less likely to form harmful substances. It is best to use extra virgin olive oil for this purpose though, as the other types of olive oil are refined.

Coconut butter is an alternative to olive oil. Unlike saturated fats from ordinary butter and meats, which contain long-chain saturated fat, coconut butter contains only short-chain saturated fat, which is not associated with health problems such as an increased risk of heart disease.

The third main type of fat is the polyunsaturated variety (PFA's). PFA's consist of molecules where hydrogen atoms are not attached. This means that they are very unstable and are readily damaged by heat, light and even when exposed to the oxygen in the air. Of course this makes a mockery of the claims made by manufacturers of such oils; namely, that they can be used for deep frying and general cooking purposes. When these oils become damaged by high heat they are harmful to the human body and they then compete with good fats for absorption into the cells.

Having said this, when PFA's are extracted using the so-called cold pressing method, rather than in cheaper processed oils, and then quickly transferred to air-tight containers which exclude light, they have health properties. Such oils can be used to make salad dressings as they are a good source of healthy fats, the most well-known of which are Omega 3 and 6 polyunsaturated fatty acids.

Omega 3 and Omega 6 Fatty Acids – Why All the Fuss?

Omega 3 and Omega 6 – the essential fatty acids or EFA's – play a key role in maintaining health. They influence healthy brain function, they lower LDL (bad) cholesterol, reduce inflammation and they have been shown to balance out behavior in children with behavioral problems, when given as a supplement or added to their diet.

These healthy fats often work in harmony with key vitamins and minerals to exert a positive affect on brain function. This was brought home to me a few years ago when I was treating a teenager with attention deficit and hyperactivity disorder (ADHD). Such children often find it difficult to concentrate and many exhibit behavioral problems, especially in school where they have to deal with the constraints of the classroom and the demands of interacting with large numbers of other children in a school setting.

This particular teenager had been excluded from school and had to have a home tutor in order to continue with his education. His diet was very poor and he was suffering from a number of nutritional deficiencies; not just vitamins, but a lack of healthy fats.

When his diet was sorted out, his concentration and behavior improved markedly. His home tutor observed that he was a lot more manageable during lessons. He had been on an improved diet and nutritional supplements which included EFA's during this time. Interestingly, when these supplements were discontinued a few months down the line, he rapidly reverted to his previous difficult behavior and poor concentration. Needless to say, his parents quickly realized what was happening and re-introduced the supplements and his condition improved as before.

Getting the Balance Right

When it comes to consumption of the omega 3 and omega 6 fatty acids, it is important to get the balance right, especially as they have very different functions in the body.

The problem we have with modern diets is that there are fewer sources of omega 3 fats compared to omega 6. This is largely due to the fact that omega 6 fats are mainly derived from seed oils, such as sunflower, soy and safflower, which are used in cooking (as already observed) and in the production of margarine spreads. In addition to this, they are also present in many processed foods. In stark contrast, omega 3 fats come from oily fish in the form of EPA (eicosapentaenoic acid) or DHA (docosahexaenoic acid).

These are used directly by the body as the building blocks of hormones that control immune function, cell growth, blood clotting and inflammation as well as being important for maintaining healthy cell membranes. Vegetarian sources of omega 3 include walnuts and flaxseeds, which then have to undergo a conversion process by the body in order make EPA and DHA.

The important thing to remember is that hormones derived from omega 3 and omega 6 fatty acids have more or less opposite effects. Those from omega 6 fatty acids tend to increase inflammation (which is an important function of the immune system), blood clotting and cell multiplication; whilst those fatty acids from omega 3 decrease those functions.

Many nutritionists now believe that before the advent of processed foods, we used to consume omega 3 and 6 fatty acids in roughly equal amounts. So it is important that your child has oily fish like sardines or salmon in their diet at least a couple of times each week. It is also beneficial to include the likes of walnuts, hulled hempseeds, flaxseeds and sesame seeds in the diet. Flaxseeds can be ground up and sprinkled onto yoghurts or on breakfast cereals.

How Much Fat Should Our Children Eat?

It's worth considering that almost all foods that contain fat have a balance of the main groups of fatty acids. For example, meat is mainly composed of saturated fat, monounsaturated fat and a little polyunsaturated fat. Oils from seeds such as sunflower contain mainly polyunsaturated fat and olive oil is composed of mostly monounsaturated fat.

As more and more children are eating fat-laden foods like burgers, chips, cheese, crisps and chocolate, their overall consumption is also way too high. The current average of fat consumption in the UK, amounts to 40%. In the USA it is even higher. Even more concerning is the fact that these types of foods contain mostly unhealthy fats. In other words, most children in Western societies are consuming saturated fats and trans-fatty acids at the expense of the health-giving fats.

You probably won't be surprised to know that the overall fat consumption in the Western world is far higher than in countries such as Japan and Thailand. Not surprisingly, since they only consume around 15% of their total calorie intake as fat, these countries have a low incidence of fat-related diseases.

Most authorities seem to agree that up to 20% of our total calorie intake should be as fat. This intake should consist of approximately up to a third of saturated fat; one third as monounsaturated fat and one third as polyunsaturated fat.

Making the Changes

Now that we are aware of the inadequacies of the Western style of diet in terms of supplying healthy fats, it is obvious that we owe it to our children to do something about it. By incorporating some or all of the following Omega 3 and Omega 6-rich foods into your child's diet, you will not only be giving them a brilliant start in life, but also laying the foundations for their future health.

Foods that Supply Omega 3 Fats

Best food sources include chia seeds, flaxseeds (linseeds), pumpkin seeds, hemp seeds, walnuts, oily fish (e.g. salmon, sardines and mackerel) and eggs.

A Special Word About Chia Seeds

Just a few months ago chia seeds would not have featured in the foregoing list of foods that supply Omega 3 fats. That's simply because I hadn't heard of them. However, I have since discovered that they are an even better source of Omega 3 fatty acids than flaxseeds.

These seeds used to be a staple food of the ancient Aztecs. However, they became a forgotten crop for 500 years, until being recently re-discovered.

The good news is that they are quickly gaining a reputation as a wonderful health food as well as a truly exceptional source of antioxidants and Omega 3 fatty acids. In fact, it is because they are so high in antioxidants that they do not deteriorate for long periods of time. This is because the antioxidants protect the unstable essential fatty acids from oxidative damage (damage by exposure to oxygen).

This is in contrast with flaxseeds, which can be damaged in the grinding process due to the heat being generated. Latest research has suggested that ground flaxseeds may only last up to 72 hours before the Omega 3 fats are damaged. So either sprinkle them whole on cereal or grind your own flaxseeds and give them to your child for immediate consumption.

In addition to a very high antioxidant level, chia seeds are an excellent source of minerals, protein, fiber, and calcium, which is worth remembering for children on dairy-free diets. Chia seeds are also an excellent source of the mineral boron, which helps to assimilate calcium.

Chia seeds have been approved as a safe food by the FDA in the USA. The only cautionary note is for people who take blood thinning medication, as the high Omega 3 fats are naturally blood thinning, the effects would therefore be increased to unacceptable levels.

N.B. For information on the best sources for chia seeds, see under Useful Information at the end of this book.

In pregnancy

Pregnant women particularly those with any health conditions, should seek advice from their doctor or natural health provider regarding the quantity of flaxseed oil they need to consume during their pregnancy. Taken within the recommended levels it should provide a beneficial supply of Omega 3 fats for healthy development of the baby.

Foods that Supply Omega 6 Fats

These include sunflower seeds, sesame seeds, pumpkin seeds, soy beans, maize and wheat-germ.

Supplements for Kids

In my role as a nutritional practitioner and advisor, I sometimes encounter parents who have tried to encourage their child to eat the omega-rich foods, but then end up frustrated because they refuse to eat them. If you find yourself in this situation, don't despair because you can use supplements. There are numerous bottled oils and capsules on the market, however, whatever you choose, it is best to opt for products that are manufactured by reputable companies that extract the oils by cold pressing. You will know if you are choosing the right product if the oil has been extracted without it being exposed to heat (cold pressing), light and air. This is important since these oils are very easily damaged by oxygen, light and heat. A good manufacturer will also use dark colored bottles in order to protect the essential fats from the light; they should also be stored in a refrigerator. Several reputable health supplement companies produce good bottled omega oils for children.

These oils can be added to the likes of yoghurts and cooked dishes at the point when they are about to be served. Alternatively, you can purchase them in capsule form, providing that your child doesn't have a problem with swallowing capsules. It would probably be wise to use the bottled oil for very young children in order to avoid swallowing hazards. You can disguise these oils by adding them to dishes, for example, to a casserole dish, or mashed potato just prior to serving. The heat from the dish will not be high enough at this stage to damage the fats.

Another advantage associated with using bottled oils is that they are suitable for children following a vegan and vegetarian diet, as they are derived purely from plant sources such as flaxseed. In addition, there are some very good fish oil supplements that comprise of oils that have had any contaminants (such as mercury) filtered out.

Warning

When pregnant do not take fish oils that are derived from fish livers as they are high in vitamin A. Too much vitamin A can cause damage to the fetus. If in doubt consult your doctor or midwife.

Fat Facts -Your Easy Reference Guide

The following easy reference guide should make it easy to distinguish between the different types of fats, when it comes to knowing which ones to buy from a health perspective.

Saturated fat in food

Coconut oil

Coconut

Palm oil

Palm kernel oil

Cocoa butter

Butter

Low-fat cheese

Chocolate

Lard

Beef

Chicken

Turkey

Hydrogenated fat

Whole milk/cream

Cheeses

Guide to polyunsaturated fats in foods

Safflower oil

Sunflower oil

Soybean oil

Rapeseed oil

Corn oil

Walnut oil
Sesame oil
Soybeans
Tofu
Margarine
Salad dressings
Nuts
Seeds

Guide to monounsaturated fats in foods
Olive oil
Olives
Coconut oil
Canola oil
Canola seeds
Avocado oil
Avocados
Peanut oil
Peanuts
Peanut butter
Cashew nuts

Key points

- Reduce the amount of saturated fats in your child's diet (meat and animal fats, and processed hydrogenated oils in processed manufactured foods).

- Try to eliminate consumption of hydrogenated fats as far as possible.

- Do make use of the nuts and seeds mentioned in this chapter.

- Use only extra virgin olive oil or coconut oil for frying and cooking.

- Purchase supplements that are manufactured by reputable companies.

- Use a little butter for spreading. Used in moderation it is actually healthier than most margarine, since the latter often contains damaged fats.

- The best margarines are those made with cold pressed oils that have not been processed.

- Use nut and seed butters as healthy alternative spreads. For example pumpkin seed butter provides a reasonable balance between Omega 3 and Omega 6 fats. Explore what is available from your local health food store or super-market. Some manufacturers offer a raw version (i.e. not roasted), which is good since the fats are not damaged by the roasting process.

Incorporate into your child's diet cold pressed unprocessed oils which are blended in order to provide a good balance between Omega 3 and Omega 6 fatty acids. These oils can be used to make a salad dressing, or can be added to foods such as yoghurts and cooked dishes that are ready to serve.

6

Label Alert!

Because parents are now becoming more educated about what goes into everyday foods, I get a lot of questions about food labels. Occasionally I receive a mobile phone call from an anxious client or parent. This isn't your average call because they are phoning me from their local supermarket whilst meticulously scanning the contents of a can of soup, or a box of breakfast cereal, or whatever. Usually the conversation goes something like this:

Parent: Hi Dave, I hope you don't mind me giving you a quick call, but you did say to get in touch if I had any questions.

Me: That's fine, how can I help?

Parent: Well, you are going to think this is crazy, but guess where I'm phoning you from?

Me: Er, the supermarket?

Parent: Blimey, how did you know?

Me: Just a lucky guess I suppose.

Parent: Well, just a quick question. I'm looking at this loaf of bread, I think it's whole wheat but it's a granary version. It says on the label it's made from wheat flour, malt extract, etc, etc. Is it ok?

Me: No, it isn't whole wheat. It just sounds healthy because the manufacturers use the word wheat flour instead of white flour, but it means the same thing.

Parent: You mean it's really white bread colored brown with a few grains in it?

Me: Correct. The malt extract colors it brown so it looks like whole wheat but it isn't.

Parent: Good grief! I've been buying granary bread for ages thinking it was whole wheat.

This kind of scenario is quite common these days because finding one's way around the label jungle is a bit of a nightmare. The problem is that manufacturers can be crafty when it comes to their labeling. You see, they often want to give us the impression that their product is healthy, when really it is quite the opposite. Remember, despite claims to the contrary, the majority of manufacturers are not usually in the business of putting our health at the top of their agenda, despite clever advertising that tries to convince us otherwise.

Guidelines for Selecting Healthy Foods

The following list will help you to discern the good from the bad when scrutinizing product labels:

- Wheat flour: This is just another name for white flour. By using the word wheat instead of white flour, it fools some shoppers into thinking it is whole wheat.

- Organic wheat flour: Again, this is just white flour. Just because it is derived from wheat that has been grown organically does not mean it is healthy.

- Sucrose: This is just the scientific name for white or brown sugar, which should be avoided.

- White sugar: Speaks for itself.

- Cane sugar: Just another name for white sugar. Remember, if it says organic cane sugar it is still refined sugar.

- Sugar syrup: Guess what? Yes, that's right; this is just a liquid version of the white stuff.

- Brown sugar: Just because it is brown doesn't mean that it is healthy. Brown sugar comes in different shades according to how refined it is. The crudest types such as dark Muscavado and molasses do contain some nutrients, and are a little better for us; but they are still not a desirable food, since they will still quickly elevate blood sugar levels.

- High fructose corn syrup, maltose, glucose, dextrose, lactose, fructose, are all simple sugars and therefore elevate blood sugar levels.

- Granary bread: As mentioned above, this is just white bread that is colored brown. It will quickly elevate blood sugar levels just like any other refined carbohydrate. Having said this, I have occasionally come across whole grain versions in health food shops, but you need to look at the labels to make sure.

- MSG (monosodium glutamate): This is an additive that is added to a multitude of foods these days which is used as a flavor-enhancer. It is a well-known ingredient in Chinese meals. It is commonly found in many savory snacks that are popular with children. It is implicated in a number of health conditions, including a possible cause of migraines in some people; so my advice would be to avoid feeding your children with monosodium glutamate whenever possible. It is possible to purchase savory snacks that have been flavored with natural flavorings. These are often available from your local health food store, or the healthy section in your supermarket.

- Aspartame: This artificial sweetener is implicated in a number of health conditions including PMS and depression.

- Hydrogenated oil or partially hydrogenated oil: This is known as a trans fat which is unnatural to the body (see Chapter 5). It also competes with good fats for absorption in the body and is linked with heart disease.

- Artificial colors: These are used to artificially color foods and confectionary in order to make them look more attractive. They can be found in a wide range of foods, so be on your guard. I'm sure you wouldn't dream of putting artificial dyes into your child's food at home when preparing meals, so my advice is to avoid these like the plague.

- Artificial flavors: These are chemical additives that are designed to get your children hooked. Like artificial colors, they are often linked with health problems, including mood swings and hyperactivity in children.

- G.M. Foods: Genetically modified foods are made from plants that have had their DNA changed in order to create certain characteristics, such as longer shelf-life or more disease-resistant crops. However, most people are concerned about their possible long-term effects on health and choose to avoid them. Unless you are happy for your children to be human guinea pigs, then I would advise you to avoid them. If in doubt about whether a food contains GM grown ingredients, contact the supermarket's customer services department and ask them to check this and confirm.

- Artificial preservatives: As the name suggests, these are designed to preserve food, thus extending its shelf-life. They work because they kill the micro-organisms that thrive on food, for example moulds and certain bacteria. Logic dictates that if they will destroy these life-forms then they can't be good for the cells in our bodies. Watch out for the likes of sodium benzoate, which is a commonly used preservative.

- Sodium nitrite: This is an additive that is added to the likes of bacon and sliced meats such as ham and frankfurters. It is used in meats like ham in order to impart an attractive red color. Studies have indicated that it forms a type of chemical in the stomach known as nitrosamines. These are known to be carcinogenic. My advice is to avoid them. When I inform parents about nitrites they are shocked that they present a health risk, as they have frequently opted for ham sandwiches for their child's packed lunches.

- Raising agents: Used for baking; avoid the ones that contain aluminum, since it has been associated with Alzheimer's disease. For the same reason you are advised to avoid using cooking utensils that are made from aluminum.

- Glazing agents: These are used to impart a shiny coating, such as wax on oranges and lemons. Select non-waxed fruit whenever possible.

FOOD FACT

These are some of the ingredients that may be found in a typical bread bun and French fries, often available from fast-food restaurants:

bread bun: enriched flour, high fructose corn syrup, sugar, yeast, soybean oil, hydrogenated or partially hydrogenated vegetable oil and less than 2% of additives that may include calcium sulfate, ammonium sulfate, calcium carbonate, dough conditioners (ascorbic acid, sodium stearoyl lactylate, azodicarbonamide), calcium peroxide, sodium propionate and calcium propionate (preservatives)

french fries may contain potatoes, canola oil, hydrgenated soy oil, natural beef flavor, citric acid (preservative), dextrose, sodium acid pyrophosphate (these maintain color), salt

---

The Cosmetic Ingredients Minefield

If you take a look at the list of ingredients used to make many cosmetic products, more often than not you will see a wide range of chemical additives, some with unpronounceable names. Some of these ingredients have been banned in other countries because their safety is in question. Some of them are thought to cause skin irritation, allergic reactions and may even be carcinogenic.

At one time, despite being careful to avoid additives in my diet, I was totally ignorant of the fact that I was using products such as shampoos and skin creams that are packed with chemical additives. This changed one day when someone who had studied the subject said to me: "Dave, you don't eat junk foods, so why would you want to absorb junk through your skin?" Point taken!

I have since discovered that chemicals are indeed absorbed through the skin, as the skin is an organ and it is a semi-permeable layer. This is aptly demonstrated when we consider that if we rub a clove of garlic on the soles of our feet we can later smell garlic on our breath.

Now, I'm not saying that parents have to become obsessed about avoiding every product on the market. But I think that it pays to be discerning; so I would advise you to look out for the worst additives and try to purchase products that use safer alternatives.

Many cosmetics and toiletries which do not contain these harmful chemicals are sold in health food shops. For a list of reputable manufacturers that use pure natural ingredients please refer to Useful Information at the end of this book.

The foregoing list of additives represent a general guide only; however, should you wish to delve into the subject further I would recommend that you purchase a book on the subject and use it as a quick reference guide, particularly if you are unsure about an ingredient. This is especially useful for parents who suspect their child is sensitive to certain additives; for example, artificial colors and flavors. A book that I particularly recommend is **The Chemical Maze** by Bill Statham (Summersdale Publishers Ltd; www.summersdale.com). This is a very comprehensive pocket-sized guide to the vast array of additives used in foods and cosmetics.

Shown below is a typical example of a list of ingredients shown on some chocolate spread. As you might imagine it contains a number of undesirable ingredients; using the guide on additives, can you spot which ones to avoid?

INGREDIENTS IN A CHOCOLATE SPREAD
Hydrogenated vegetable fat, sugar, lactose, fat-reduced cocoa, skimmed milk powder, emulsifier (soy lecithin), vitamins (B1, B2, B12, E), flavorings

---

7

Allergic Kids

What is an Allergy?

An allergy occurs when the body becomes over-sensitive to a food or an external substance. For example, when we eat a food that we are sensitive to, the immune system over-reacts to its presence in the body. In other words it is an exaggerated defensive reaction by the body to something that is normally harmless.

When this happens the body's natural defensive reaction is to release a substance called histamine from cells known as mast cells. It is this histamine that causes inflammation in the tissues, resulting in the classic symptoms of immediate gastro-intestinal discomfort, rhinitis, hay fever, skin rashes, eczema, sinusitis and asthma.

With this kind of reaction it is easier to isolate the food or substance that has invoked the reaction, since the immune system is quick to over-react. An extreme example would be anaphylactic shock, which can occur as a result of an allergy to certain foods, for example, certain nuts, especially peanuts.

This type of reaction by the body can be life-threatening, and we sometimes read in the news that someone has died due to anaphylactic shock as a result of exposure to a minute amount of a substance; for example, a trace of peanut oil in a meal. Or, it might occur as a result of a bee or wasp sting, when the body over-reacts to the poison from the bee or wasp. Thankfully, this kind of scenario is not common; however, it would appear that allergies are on the increase; including food allergies.

The Mechanism Behind Allergies and Intolerancies

The immune system is the body's defense system. When it

encounters something it doesn't like it produces 'markers'. These markers are known as antibodies called IgE (immunoglobulin type E). The antibodies attach themselves to 'mast cells'.

When an offending substance (e.g. a food) called an allergen, combines with its specific IgE marker (antibody), the resulting IgE antibody triggers the mast cell to release histamine and other chemicals normally associated with causing the typical allergic reactions.

I am frequently asked by parents why allergies to every day foods are more prevalent these days. My observations have led me to conclude that allergies are an illness which is associated with our Western style of living.

Undoubtedly we are all exposed to chemicals in the form of pesticides, fungicides and artificial nitrates from commercially-grown fruits, vegetables and grains. In addition, most people eat too many refined, packaged and adulterated foods that contain too much salt and are laced with chemical additives. These foods are also high in unhealthy fats and are lacking in vital nutrients. Many of us base our diet largely around excessive amounts of wheat and wheat products, which may be largely responsible for the rapid increase in gluten sensitivity. And on top of that, we are all exposed to a vast array of chemical substances in our environment that were unheard of just a few decades ago. Is it any wonder, therefore, that the immune system becomes compromised, resulting in a greater propensity towards developing sensitivities, intolerances and allergies?

Intolerances

Some reactions to food do not involve IgE antibodies. These are sometimes referred to as intolerances or sensitivities. They are different from the quick reactions associated with IgE antibodies, and may take hours or even days to show up. It is probable that these delayed reactions are linked with another type of marker known as IgG. antibodies. These also attach themselves to allergens, but they only manifest allergic symptoms when they reach a certain level in the body.

In my experience as a nutritional practitioner I have come across many people who suffer from a wide range of food intolerances, including an increasing number of children. Even babies can begin to manifest problems early, especially when introduced to cow's milk.

I am often asked which intolerances occur most frequently and I have no hesitation in stating that grains and diary come top of the list. With regard to grains, I come across a lot of wheat intolerance as well as intolerance to gluten, which is a protein component of wheat (including spelt), barley, rye and oats.

The health problems that food intolerances can cause are diverse, and the same intolerance to a specific food may manifest itself in different ways in different people. Some of the conditions that both adults and children with food intolerances suffer from include eczema, skin rashes, digestive problems, weight gain, arthritis, depression, headaches, 'fuzzy headiness', excessive tiredness, frequent infections, irritable bowel syndrome (IBS), constipation, behavioral problems, poor concentration and hyperactivity (this is more common in children).

Excluding the offending food or foods from the diet often results in complete recovery from the associated health problem. For example, I recently encountered an 18 month old baby that was suffering from an eczema-like condition all over its body. This child was in a great degree of discomfort because the condition made him feel itchy all over. A food intolerance test identified sensitivity to gluten, and when this was removed from his diet he made a remarkable recovery in just one week. I also recall a teenage girl who had a gluten intolerance identified. She had suffered from irritable bowel syndrome for months and had been to see different consultants. They could do nothing to solve her problem; however, once she omitted gluten from her diet, her symptoms gradually disappeared. She was also delighted to experience an improvement in regulating her weight, which had been a problem for some time. I have witnessed similar results with many other people over the years.

What to Do if You Suspect Your Child Has a Food Intolerance

There are a number of allergy tests available. I have worked with bio-impedance testing for a number of years and have found it to be quite reliable for detecting food intolerances and other sensitivities, (e.g. pollen and dust mite intolerances). However, it is important to ensure that the practitioner carrying out the testing is proficient, since varied results may otherwise ensue.

The big advantage with this type of testing is that it is non-invasive and you receive the results immediately. It works by measuring electrical resistance in the body's energy channels known as meridians, which were identified by the Chinese hundreds of years ago. The technology was invented by Reinhold Voll, a German medical doctor in the 1950's.

Patrick Holford, one of the world's leading nutritionists and founder of the Institute Of Optimum Nutrition in the UK, recommends the IgG ELISA test. This involves taking a small blood sample using a home test kit. A special device painlessly pricks your finger and the blood that is produced enters a tiny tube. You then send this to the laboratory where it is tested. The good news is that this type of test not only tests for any foods that you may be sensitive to, but also how strong your allergic reaction is. This is very useful because it is possible to suffer from one or more dominant sensitivities, whilst other less dominant types may still be affecting your child.

Once you are aware of which foods your child should avoid, then you can plan a diet which excludes them. Patrick Holford regards this test as being very reliable. In the UK, a company called YorkTest provide a home testing service (see under 'Useful Information at the end of this book). You simply take a pin-prick of blood and send it back to them in a pre-paid package. The results are available in about seven to ten days. They also offer consultation with one of their nutritionists in order to discuss your results.

Important! YorkTest do not conduct tests for children under two years of age without a doctor's referral. This is because the digestive system in children under two has not developed sufficiently enough to digest some foods.

Residents from other countries such as Australia and the USA will have access to similar testing services (see under 'Useful Information').

Leaky Gut Syndrome

This is a condition which is produced when the lining of the gut becomes inflamed, perhaps due to intolerance, the excessive use of antibiotics or a 'junk' food diet. As the name suggests, the gut becomes permeable and partly digested proteins can then pass through the gut-wall and into the blood stream. These proteins are suspected by some nutritionists as being responsible for triggering allergic reactions. However, the good news is that the gut can be healed and food sensitivities reduced. The following methods can be employed in order to achieve this:

- Consistent with the advice in this book, base your child's diet largely upon natural foods such as fruits, vegetables, nuts, seeds and whole-grains.

- Avoid any foods that he/she is sensitive to.

- Supplement the diet with so-called friendly bacteria, otherwise known as probiotics. Refer to 'Useful Information' at the end of the book for reputable companies that produce probiotic formulas for children.

- Use a supplement that contains a fatty acid known as butyric acid. This substance helps to heal the gut wall. A few grams of glutamine powder in water or fruit juice taken a few hours away from food can also help to heal a leaky gut.

How to Reduce Your Child's Allergic Potential

As with leaky gut syndrome, try to feed your child on a natural diet and avoid any foods that you are aware he/she is sensitive to. In addition, attempt to implement the following measures:

Grains

Wheat is the most commonly used grain in Western society. It is used to make bread, bakery goods such as cakes and biscuits, pies, sausage rolls, quiches, spaghetti, pasta and noodles. In addition to this, wheat flour is added to many foods such as packaged and tinned soups, confectionary, savory snacks and many more items.

I believe that heavy exposure to wheat in its variety of forms is partly responsible for the development of wheat and gluten sensitivities. In addition to this, modern wheat is very different from early types of wheat which was naturally lower in gluten content and was grown without the use of pesticides and artificial fertilizers.

In order to reduce your child's chances of developing an allergy or intolerance to wheat or gluten, it wise to try and make good use of products made with other grains.

For example, rye-bread, rice cakes, oat-cakes and bread made from spelt wheat which is naturally lower in gluten. There are also lots of different breakfast cereal alternatives available from health food shops, and to some degree in supermarkets. For instance, you can introduce your child to rice puffs that are made from whole-grain rice. You can also try products such as pasta and spaghetti that are made from gluten-free and wheat-free alternatives. You might need to try a few of these products in order to find the ones that are palatable to your child. If you can get children to develop a taste for these foods, particularly when very young, then you may be saving them from developing allergies and intolerances in the future.

Examples of wheat-free and gluten-free foods

NB. Remember that if a food or product is gluten-free, it is automatically wheat-free, since you can't have wheat in a gluten-free product.

Quinoa (pronounced keen-wa)

Consisting of small round grains, quinoa originates from South America, where it was once considered "the gold of the Incas". When we delve into its nutritional make up we can see why it was so highly revered, since it is very high in protein compared to other grains. Moreover, it is a good source of the minerals, manganese, magnesium and iron.

As far as its culinary benefits are concerned, quinoa is very versatile. For example, it can be used as a substitute for cous cous, made into porridge, for a great energizing start to the day; and added to salads, much like rice. Quinoa can also be used to make bakery products such as cakes and biscuits, and when added to other flours, such as rice flour, it is sometimes used to make gluten-free bread.

Rice

Rice is regarded as an extremely healthy food, partly because rice allergy is less likely compared to most other grains. Whole grain rice is a good source of energy from its starch content, as well as being high in important fiber. This is in stark contrast to white rice which is lacking in the important rice-bran (fiber) and rice 'germ', which contains most of its nutrients. For this reason, it is advisable to try and get children used to eating the healthier whole grain versions of rice. I say versions, because we sometimes forget that there are many different forms of rice, including long grain, short grain, basmati and wild rice. So make good use of the different varieties as much as possible. It's good to try and get your child used to eating the different types of whole grain rice; otherwise they will only accept the refined white version.

From a culinary point of view, rice can be used to make risotto, added to casseroles, eaten as an accompaniment to other dishes, such as curries, and even used to make lovely rice puddings. What's more, rice cakes made from whole grain rice are a gluten-free substitute for wheat crackers and bread.

Rice flour is often used as an ingredient in gluten-free bread, in addition to being used to make rice noodles and other gluten-free products. It is also a very fine light flour, perfect for baking cakes.

Warning! Recent research has indicated that some rice products, including whole grain rice and rice milk, contain higher levels of inorganic arsenic. Rice from certain geographical regions are higher than others, for example, rice from Bangladesh and USA (especially long grain rice). Sourcing low arsenic contaminated rice would be wise; for example some information suggests that rice grown in Egypt and China may be less contaminated. However, further research is needed. Babies and toddlers who consume rice milk may be more at risk.

Corn

Corn is one of those ancient grains that has been used by different cultures, including the Native Americans, over hundreds of years. It is referred to scientifically as Zea mays, which reflects its traditional name, maize. As well as being regarded as a cereal crop, corn is sold as a vegetable in the form of corn on the cob, a firm favorite with most kids. However, it is an extremely versatile food which is also a good source of carbohydrate, fiber and nutrients, such as beta carotene, niacin (a B vitamin needed by the digestive system and nerves), potassium and vitamin C.

Corn is ground into corn flour, which is used in many products, including some gluten-free bread and other bakery goods. It is also made into corn chips, gluten-free pasta, corn flakes and popcorn. Corn crisp bread is usually made from 100% corn and is an alternative to rice cakes.

Buckwheat

Despite its name, buckwheat is not related to wheat in any way. In fact, it isn't even a grain, but rather a fruit seed that is related to rhubarb and the plant, sorrel. Nutritionally, it is a great source of health-promoting and protective compounds called flavonoids, especially rutin. These flavonoids are beneficial for the cardiovascular system by promoting good blood flow and reducing bad cholesterol, known as LDL, or low density lipoproteins.

It is also exceptionally high in the mineral magnesium, which many people are deficient in these days. Magnesium is essential for good health as it is involved in hundreds of biochemical reactions in the body, as well as being crucial for energy production, bone formation and many other processes.

Having said this, if your child is eating natural, health-giving foods, as advocated in this book, he or she will normally be getting enough of this crucial mineral.

Buckwheat is a great alternative food for those on wheat and gluten-free diets. It is used to make buckwheat noodles and is a common ingredient in specialized breakfast cereals and bakery products such as gluten-free bread. In the USA, buckwheat pancakes made with buckwheat flour and served with maple syrup, are a popular dessert.

Millet

Millet is another one of those ancient grains and in Biblical times it was used to make bread. It was also used as a staple food in Africa and Asia for hundreds of years. It is also part of the staple diet of the Hunzas, who use it to make a type of bread called a chapatti. In India, it is traditionally used to make thin flat cakes called roti.

From a nutritional point of view millet is highly nutritious and easy to digest. It contains plenty of fiber, B vitamins, the essential amino-acid, methionine (which the body cannot manufacture), lecithin, vitamin E, iron, magnesium, potassium, phosphorous and is almost 15% protein. Moreover, unlike most grains, it is alkaline-forming, making it mild on the digestion and the body.

Millet can be cooked much like rice, and it is suggested that you use 3 parts water to 1 part millet. It is advisable to add the grain to boiling water, and then simmer until the water is thoroughly absorbed. You can also use stock in place of the water. Try using it in soups, casseroles, stews and to make bakery products such as breads and cakes.

In common with other grains, such as quinoa, you can even sprout millet grains and use them in salads and sandwiches. Millet flakes are often used in gluten and wheat-free breakfast cereals, such as muesli.

Amaranth

Amaranth is one of those lesser known grains. However, as interest in looking for alternatives to wheat grows amongst the population, amaranth is slowly being recognized as a nutritious and versatile grain.

Amaranth was part of the staple diet of the Aztecs and to this day it is used by a variety of different cultures. For example, in Mexico it is used to make a drink called "atole". In Nepal, the seeds are made into flour and used to make chapattis.

From a nutritional perspective, amaranth consists of up to 18% protein, in addition to containing two essential amino acids, methionine and lysine, which are uncommon in most grains. It is also a good source of fiber, vitamins A and C, and the minerals iron, calcium and potassium. Combined with other grains, such as corn and rice, it provides a complete protein with all of the amino acids needed by the body.

In common with the other gluten-free grains, amaranth is versatile. You can cook it as a cereal, add it to casseroles, soups, salads and stews; and the flour is sometimes used to make bakery products such as breads and pastas. When making breads, it is often added to other gluten-free flours such as rice and corn. Also, it is often used in gluten and wheat-free breakfast cereals.

Teff
It does seem, doesn't it, that all non-gluten grains are ancient ones? Certainly Teff is no exception, since it appears that it originated in Ethiopia thousands of years ago. Teff is unusual in that it is the smallest grain in the world, and it takes around 150 grains to equal 1 wheat grain.

In common with other grains, Teff consists of bran, starch (carbohydrate) and the nutrient rich germ. It is a good source of nutrients such as phosphorous, copper, iron, protein and the B vitamin thiamin. It also has a good amino acid profile with higher levels of lysine compared to some other grains such as wheat.

When ground into flour, it can be used to make grain burgers, porridge, puddings and added as a thickener to soups, stews and casseroles. It is also used to brew alcoholic beverages.

When cooking Teff, you use 2 cups of water with ½ cup of the grain. Bring to the boil in a saucepan, then simmer until most of the water is absorbed. The grains can also be sprouted and added to salads and used in sandwiches.

Non grain options

Many parents are worried that their child may be missing out on carbohydrates when wheat and gluten is omitted from the diet. However, as we have seen with the gluten-free grains, they are an equally good source of carbohydrate in the form of starch. Having said this, there are other foods unrelated to grains that provide us with carbohydrates. For example, pulses such as peas, beans, lentils and chick-peas are an excellent source of both protein and starch. Not only this, unlike foods like potatoes, and some grains, pulses do not cause a rapid rise in blood glucose levels. This makes them excellent for children and adults suffering from Type 2 diabetes or those suffering from hypoglycemia.

Chick peas are used a lot in Asian cooking, either whole, or ground into flour and used to make bhajis – a deep fried savory mixture of onions, chick-pea flour and spices – and poppadoms. Pulses such as peas, kidney beans and aduki beans are a great addition to casseroles, soups and stews. Lentils are used in Asian cooking to make dhal; a spicy dish. They are also used to make the likes of lentil roast – a mixture of potatoes, onions, lentils and gravy; and we are all familiar with baked beans made, with haricot beans. Of course, baked beans have the reputation of producing gas; but in that sense they are similar to most pulses. This is because the combination of starch and high protein is difficult to digest for some people. Also, most pulses contain enzyme inhibitors which interfere with protein digestion. Most of these are deactivated when the pulses are cooked thoroughly. Also, pulses become much more digestible when sprouted.

Starchy tuberous root vegetables

These are vegetables that grow under the ground and store energy in the form of starch and sugars. Good examples are yams, sweet potatoes and potatoes. They are a good addition to a gluten-free diet, especially as they are so versatile. For example, sweet potatoes can be baked, mashed and added to other dishes such as soups or stir-fries.

Squashes

This group of vegetables comes in all sorts of colors, shapes and sizes. They are often a good source of carbohydrate in the form of starch. Kid's favorites often include kabucha, onion and butternut squashes. They can be baked, added to stir-fries and used in soups and casseroles.

Strengthening Your Child's Immune System

Your child is much more likely to develop both environmental and food allergies/ or intolerances if their immune system is compromised by toxins generated by a poor diet and a polluted environment.

What's more, the situation is compounded because a diet high in refined foods is lacking in the essential nutrients that are the very building-blocks that the immune system needs to function normally.

In fact, you might be surprised to know that eating such foods actually depletes the body's reserves of nutrients in order for them to be digested in the first place. No wonder children who live on junk foods are low in energy, moody, prone to infections, and exhibit poor concentration and behavioral problems.

Probiotics

Probiotics, or beneficial bacteria such a lactobacillus acidophilus and bifido bacteria, help to create a healthy gut environment, which in turn can help to calm down a reactive digestive tract; thus reducing the occurrence of allergic responses. The healthy bacteria in the gut are often compromised these days as a result of over consumption of junk foods; particularly refined carbohy-drates, including sugar and white flour products.

Becoming Allergy-Free

Not surprisingly, it is not unusual for allergies to subside when the diet is improved. The fact is, given the right conditions, the immune system will function much better when it is supplied with the nutrients it needs to function properly. It will also function at an optimum level when it is not hampered by a high degree of toxicity within the body. Following the advice on healthy eating in the preceding chapters will do much to reduce your child's allergic potential and may help to eliminate allergies that already exist.

This is summed up in the following contrasting equations:

Junk Food = Toxins + Nutrient Deficiencies/Imbalances = Weakened Immune System = Allergies/Intolerances

Natural Food = Less Toxicity + Higher Nutrient Levels = Stronger Immune System = Greater Resistance to Allergies/Intolerances

Immune Boosting Supplements

The good news is that there are a number of natural supplements available that help to strengthen your child's immune system.

Some of the most well-known supplements are:

- Echinacea – this herb is a natural antibiotic and infection fighter. It helps to kill fungi, viruses, bacteria and other harmful microbes. Its action in the body involves the stimulation of various immune-system cells that are designed to fight infection. It also helps to strengthen the immune system. I recommend it as a remedy for eczema; in fact I used this herb, along with a healthy diet, to help cure my own son of eczema when he was growing up. I would recommend that you use echinacea drops (tincture). If you add the drops to unsweetened fruit juice, such as apple, then this disguises the flavor (see chapter 13, Super Plants).

- Aloe vera – This is another herb that has an immune-boosting effect. It is most often taken in the form of aloe vera juice, but be careful to seek out a good make. Look for the IASC-certified seal, especially when purchasing the juice (see chapter 13, Super Plants).

- Children's vitamin and mineral formulae – A good vitamin and mineral formula can be used in conjunction with a healthy diet in order to strengthen the immune system. Avoid poor quality makes, especially those that contain sugar, artificial sweeteners and other artificial additives. Select brands made by reputable manufacturers, such as Higher Nature, Solgar, Lambert's and Biocare. These are produced more healthily than many commercial brand vitamins available in drug stores. Higher Nature produces a naturally-flavored chewable tablet called Dinochews. The dosage is related to the age of the child.

Important! Do not exceed the manufacturers recommended dosages of vitamins for children.

Summary:
In order to strengthen your child's resistance to allergies/intolerances you need to do the following:

1. Exclude junk foods in the diet.
2. Minimize processed foods in the diet.
3. Base the diet largely around natural unprocessed foods.
4. Make use of a variety of whole grains and the other gluten and wheat-free alternatives, not just refined wheat and wheat-based products.

5. Consider giving your child additional immune-boosting and immune regulating supplements.

What About Severe Allergies?

Those children with severe allergies that could lead to anaphylactic shock – a potentially life-threatening condition – will need specialist treatment. Currently, studies in the USA and the UK are taking place with children who suffer from severe peanut allergy. They are using an approach called desensitization therapy, which involves exposing an allergic child to minute amounts of peanut on a daily basis. One such study at Duke University Medical Center and Arkansas Children's Hospital in the USA, has produced very good results. Such exposure has resulted in positive changes in the children's immune systems, leading to long-term tolerance to the peanuts. MD, Wesley Burks, Chief of the Division of Pediatric Allergy and Immunology at Duke has this to say about the study:

"At the start of the study, these participants couldn't tolerate one-sixth of a peanut". He also stated: "Six months into it, they were ingesting 13 to 15 peanuts before they had a reaction".

A similar trial was conducted at Cambridge's Addenbrooke's Hospital in the UK, where they had equal success. The hope is that this approach may prove equally effective with other food allergies.

Warning! It is important that parents do not attempt to carry out this type of experiment at home with their own child, as it would be potentially dangerous. This is because a child may react and need emergency treatment. If your child has a severe allergy I would suggest that you make enquiries about desensitization therapy in your locality.

FAQ's on the Subject of Allergies and Food Intolerances

- I have just tested positive for wheat intolerance. Can I eat spelt?

Answer: No, since spelt is a type of wheat.

- My child has intolerance to gluten. Is there a chance that he might grow out of it?

Answer: Yes, it's possible that he could grow out of his gluten intolerance. Some people find that if it is omitted from the diet for, let's say 12 months, they can tolerate gluten containing grains in small amounts. However, not everyone is so lucky since some gluten sensitive adults/children have to avoid it for life.

- My daughter suffers from really bad congested sinuses, especially in the mornings when she wakes up. Could this be connected with food intolerance?

Answer: Sometimes mucous congestion is due to a diet which contains too many mucous-forming foods, such as cheese, milk and yoghurts. In such instances it is important to reduce or eliminate consumption of these foods in order to eliminate the problem. On the other hand, as you suggest, food intolerance could be at the root of the problem. I have known children who were tested positive for wheat, or gluten and having omitted these from their diet, their sinus congestion completely cleared in a matter of weeks. This kind of response can occur, irrespective of the food one is intolerant to.

- My teenage son has a lot of trouble in regulating his weight, even though he engages in a lot of sports. In fact, he is about a stone overweight. I've heard that food intolerance can result in weight regulation problems, is this true?

Answer: Yes, this is quite often the case when someone has developed sensitivity to a food, or perhaps to more than one food. This happens because the body treats the offending food as a toxin, and its way of dealing with toxins is to retain fluid in order to dilute its effects. This means, of course, that the individual concerned suffers from some degree of fluid retention. The metabolism is also adversely affected and this further adds to the weight regulation problem. A good example of this is when someone is intolerant to wheat or gluten. Once gluten is omitted from the diet the digestive system begins to heal itself, and the metabolic rate appears to improve. This, coupled with the body ridding itself of the excess fluid can only mean one thing – initial weight loss and improved weight regulation. For further information see my book on the subject: The Big Fat Mystery (Metro Books).

- I suffer from a number of food intolerances, an allergy to nuts, and I also have a respiratory sensitivity to dog hair. I am worried that I may have passed this on to my three year old daughter as she does get a bit wheezy when our pet dog is in close proximity to her. Can you suggest the best course of action in order to tackle the problem?

Answer: I have concluded that people who experience these sorts of problems have a compromised immune system. Many natural therapists subscribe to the view that when the immune system is under stress, then we are more likely to manifest problems with allergies and food intolerances.

Therefore, it stands to reason that the way to tackle this situation is to help the immune system with immune boosting natural remedies and by relieving the body of toxins. A high level of toxicity can sometimes lead to an under-functioning or malfunctioning immune system.

In this kind of scenario, it is a good idea to consult a recognized naturopath, or nutritional practitioner (see 'Useful Information' at the end of this book) who will advise you regarding the best course of treatment. A good homeopath may be able to treat your daughter constitutionally and may also help to redress hereditary factors. As for passing on these problems to your daughter; again this should be mentioned to a suitable practitioner who will advise you regarding her diet. Adhering to healthy eating habits will also help.

- My daughter had a blood test for celiac disease which proved negative. This is a real puzzle since she always gets ill when she eats gluten. Could the test results be wrong?

Answer: The blood test for celiac disease tests for the antibodies that are normally present when an allergy to gluten exists. However, it has been my experience that a person who may not be allergic to gluten can be intolerant to it. This is why someone who is intolerant to gluten may not react so severely to a small amount of gluten in the diet. In fact it may take a few hours or even a day to manifest itself in the form of symptoms. In this kind of scenario it is often advisable to have an IgG test for gluten; or be tested by a method called electro-dermal testing. (Refer to 'Food Allergy/Intolerance Testing' – under 'Useful Information' at the end of this book).

- My 12 year old son suffers from intolerance to wheat. I try not to give him wheat in his diet, but it is so difficult because it seems to be in everything. Also, he feels so deprived without it.

Answer: Admittedly, adjusting to any changes in your child's diet can be difficult at first. However, the thing to do is to try and change his attitude to the food. What I mean by this is to try to get him to focus upon all of the wonderful things that he can have instead of those he cannot. I always say to people who find themselves in your situation to imagine that they are living in a poor country where food is scarce; perhaps they would be limited to eating rice and a few vegetables on a daily basis. Then I ask them to imagine being magically transported to the middle of a typical supermarket in the UK or USA. I ask them to imagine what they would feel like when they opened their eyes, only to be confronted with this vast and wonderful array of foods.

One client said "I would think I'd died and gone to heaven!" I think that sums up the point I am making, and since children have lively imaginations, it's worth trying with them too. When I look at the amazing variety of foods provided for us by Mother Nature, I feel very grateful that there is so much choice. However, this is not to underestimate the problems that parents can encounter when trying to help their child avoid the likes of wheat, gluten and dairy. In order to educate yourself and your child about the alternatives it is always a good idea to seek out good recipe books on specialized diets.

- My son has been on a wheat-free diet three months now and he no longer suffers from excessive tiredness and bloating. He had a small amount of wheat by accident and noticed an immediate reaction. Is this normal?

Answer: Yes, I have observed this phenomenon quite a lot actually. It seems that when someone is sensitive to a food that they are having on a frequent basis, the immune system's reaction is dampened down by the frequent exposure.

However, when the body is no longer bombarded with the toxin (food) it seems to react more acutely when exposed to even a small amount.

8

No Kidding the Kids!

When I was in my twenties I became the father of two bright and healthy children. It was a magical time, and I was surprised to discover that I was very paternal. To be honest, I wasn't sure whether I would be a natural dad. I think that this probably applies to a lot of men; until you actually experience fatherhood, you don't really have a clue about how you are going to feel about bringing up your own off-spring.

Looking back, I wouldn't have swapped that experience for anything. Of course it's all a bit of a learning curve, and you sort of pick things up as you go along, so to speak. This certainly applies to feeding your children.

In my case, things were somewhat unusual. You see, I had this background in nutrition; I was clued-in about healthy eating, and although attitudes towards healthy eating in the 1980s were changing in countries like the UK, USA and Australia, it was still considered by many to be a New Age kind of thing.

However, undaunted, I set about the task of feeding my kids with as many natural foods as possible. When they were babies I would seek out the organic baby foods, and I would try to ensure that home-prepared meals were healthy. When they were in their early years this was no problem, since I was able to control things very nicely thank you; and generally speaking, our children did eat quite healthily, with a diet that was far better than average.

So far so good; until, that is, they start to get a bit older. First there are the birthday parties and tea parties. What about all those junk foods full of colorings, sugar, white flour, and goodness knows what?

Suddenly I was faced with a dilemma that every parent who is orientated towards healthy eating has to face. Do you just go with the flow and accept that they are going to be exposed to eating all of this unhealthy stuff from time to time? Or do you go along with it because you have to, but make your unease about the situation obvious to all and sundry? Unfortunately I chose the latter, and I now realize of course, that it was the worst thing I could have possibly done. In other words, when it comes to healthy eating, if parents become too purist in their approach, the wrong kind of message is conveyed to the child. They become as tense over the situation as you are, because children are very perceptive. Conflict begins to creep in because the last thing children want is to be different from their peers. This kind of scenario can result in a child rejecting the healthy eating route and choosing to eat more junk foods.

The second dilemma that I faced was that of the dreaded packed-lunch. Again, as you will imagine, I wanted to include as many healthy foods as possible. So, I would make cheese and salad sandwiches on whole wheat bread, include the little packet of raisins, the apple or carrot sticks, and maybe some natural savory snack or healthy fruit yoghurt.

This all sounds fine, and at first my children were happy enough with this situation; until the two arch-enemies creep in – boredom and competition from other children's packed lunches. The former was always a problem, because children have their own preferences, and there are only so many ways that you can include a variety of healthy foods each day.

Moreover, when it comes to sorting out the ingredients in that lunch-box, even if you set about the task with the imagination and tenacity of one of the world's health-orientated chef's, those ingredients are always going to be compared with little Johnny's white-bread ham sandwiches, packet of crisps, and chocolate bar. Pester power sets in. Oh well, nobody said this parenting business was easy!

The Benefits of Hindsight

Oh yes, hindsight is indeed a wonderful thing! If I was placed in that situation again I certainly would approach things very differently. However, as the saying goes, we sometimes have to learn from our mistakes, and on a positive note, this is why I am writing this chapter, so that you don't fall into the 'purist trap'. With this in mind, I have highlighted a number of key points that might help you to strike a balance in your quest to bring-up your child with a healthy attitude towards good nutrition:

- When it comes to planning healthy meals and packed lunches, try to bring your child into the choice. In this way they will be far more likely to eat and enjoy the food, since they have included some of their own choices.

- Accept that from time to time your child will eat some unhealthy foods. Depriving them of these kinds of foods will make them feel alienated from their peers, and they will associate those kinds of foods as being more exciting than the healthy equivalents.

- Try to educate your children about the importance of healthy eating from a young age. Use whatever literature that you think is appropriate.

- Try to introduce your child to a variety of healthy natural foods. In this way, they will develop an appreciation of lots of different flavors and textures. Children brought up in this way are far more likely to try new foods, and they will learn to appreciate the flavors in fruits and vegetables; yes, even the dreaded broccoli!

- If your child is out food shopping with you, attempt to get them involved with some of the decision-making concerning the types of healthy foods they would like to include in their meals. Allow the occasional unhealthy food or snack, such as sweets or chocolate treat. In this way your child will not feel deprived, and if they are becoming more knowledgeable about healthy eating, they are more apt to want the healthy foods that that they are developing a taste for anyway.

- Don't forget to emphasize the positive benefits of eating healthy foods, such as better concentration in lessons, less mood swings, more energy, less time feeling poorly with infections, more chance of being free from heart-disease and other killer diseases adults get in their future lives.

- If you are eating out just be as selective as possible. Try not to make it into a big issue if the choices are limited. Some restaurants will comply with your requests for healthy salads, and an increasing number cater for those with food allergies. For instance, I have discovered that some pizza restaurants (from a well-known pizza chain), offer gluten free pizzas, and others allow customers to bring in their own gluten-free or wheat-free pizza base. You just choose your own toppings and they cook it for you. Now that's what you call progress!

9

Organic Food

Pesticides on my carrot,
Nitrates in my pear,
Fungicides in my cereal,
No one seems to care;
Hormones in my chicken,
All 'fresh from the farm',
Yes, give me all my chemicals,
They won't do us kids no harm!

David Reavely – 2006

Not too many years ago, the only way that everyday folk in the UK could get hold of organically-grown produce was to seek out local farmers who didn't use chemical sprays, or maybe speak to owners of local small holdings or allotments and find out those who were growing their produce the old-fashioned way.

In fact, as a young man, that's exactly what I did in my home town (now a city) of Sunderland in the north-east of England. As far as I know, those allotments are still there, and I like to think that those local allotment holders are still producing fruits and vegetables without resorting to chemical poisons, as they were inclined to do all those years ago. Nowadays, the choice of organic produce at our disposal is huge and the demand for it is growing every year.

Of course the big question is: Why is there such a great demand for organic produce?

The answer is largely down to information and growing awareness and discernment among the general public – despite the millions spent on advertising by the processed food industry. The fact is, people are becoming more aware of the dangers associated with using many tons of chemicals in order to produce our food. Whilst many parents are too busy to think about it and decide to simply ignore the problem, an increasing number of us are not prepared for our children to be human guinea pigs. And luckily it's become much easier to be fussy; just take a look in your nearest supermarket and you'll see plenty of organically grown fruit and vegetables, organically reared free-range meat, and organic healthier food snacks for kids, as well as a wide range of organic baby foods.

There has been much controversy in the media recently suggesting that organic foods taste no different from chemically grown produce.

One recent study in July 2009, led by researchers from the London School of Hygiene and Tropical Medicine, aimed to test whether organic food is more nutritious than conventionally produced food. The researchers concluded that the difference in nutrient levels was neglible. These conclusions were contested by the Soil Association, the UK's leading and best-known organic control body, on the basis that the study was too small. Besides, the study was looking at nutrients such as protein and fat, not addressing the chemical content which is the main health reason why people choose to buy organically grown food.

Nevertheless, whether we are talking about differences in taste or nutrient levels, most of the so-called experts on the subject seem to have lost sight of the main reason consumers are buying organic foods in ever increasing numbers; namely, that they are not happy with the idea that conventionally grown foods contain a cocktail of chemicals that may have harmful affects upon themselves and their children. In fact, pesticide and fungicide residues are commonly detected on randomly selected produce on sale in countries such as the UK and USA. Proponents of conventional farming methods argue that these chemicals have to undergo stringent testing to prove their safety; however, none of the leading experts in the world can categorically state that they are safe when ingested in isolation; and especially when they occur as a combination of different chemicals derived from a variety of produce.

What if You Can't Afford to Buy Organic?

Now, having stated the case for feeding ourselves and our precious children organically grown food, I am very much aware that it is more expensive than intensively farmed food and chemically grown crops, and that there are many parents who just cannot afford to buy organic food. If you fall into this category, I would recommend that you try to prioritize and purchase at least some organic produce, such as carrots and potatoes.

Also, it is possible to be more selective when it comes to choosing which conventionally grown produce is least likely to be sprayed. Broccoli is a vegetable which is less likely to be contaminated. And avocadoes come down pretty low on the list as they seem not to require heavy use of pesticides.

It is also a good idea to choose fruits with tough skins, such as melons, since the skin helps to prevent as much of the chemical residues from penetrating into the flesh; although some will be taken up by the roots of the plant and be transported into the fruit itself, it is still better than eating the likes of grapes and strawberries which are eaten in their entirety, skin and all. In fact, grapes, peaches, strawberries and raspberries are usually heavily sprayed, so wash them before eating (peel the peaches) and do choose the organically grown ones if there is an option. If you are lucky enough to have access to an affordable organic source of them, then that is a great option as they contain many natural compounds such as antioxidants that help to keep our children healthy.

The Environmental Working Group, a non-profit making organization that aims to use the power of public information to protect public health and the environment, have produced an excellent guide for shoppers that shows the levels of pesticides in different fruits and vegetables. With their permission, I have included the guide below which shows the worst ranked foods in the left hand column:

RANK	FRUIT OR VEGGIE	SCORE
1 (worst)	Peach	100 (highest pesticide load)
2	Apple	93
3	Sweet bell pepper	83
4	Celery	82
5	Nectarine	81
6	Strawberries	80
7	Cherries	73
8	Kale	69
9	Lettuce	67
10	Grapes – Imported	66
11	Carrot	63
12	Pear	63
13	Collard greens	60
14	Spinach	58
15	Potato	56
16	Green beans	53
17	Summer squash	53
18	Red pepper/green pepper	51
19	Cucumber	50
20	Raspberries	46
21	Grapes (USA)	44
22	Plums	44
23	Orange	44
24	Cauliflower	39
25	Tangerine	37
26	Mushrooms	36

27	Banana	34
28	Winter squash	34
29	Cantaloupe	33
30	Cranberries	33
31	Honeydew Melon	30
32	Grapefruit	29
33	Sweet Potato	29
34	Tomato	29
35	Broccoli	28
36	Watermelon	26
37	Papaya	20
38	Eggplant	20
39	Cabbage	17
40	Kiwi	13
41	Peas-Frozen	10
42	Asparagus	10
43	Mango	9
44	Pineapple	7
45	Sweet Corn – Frozen	2
46	Avocado	1
47 (best)	Onion	1 (Lowest pesticide load)

Organic Box Schemes

Organic box schemes involve a local supplier of organic produce delivering fresh produce to your door. They usually have a website which allows you to see at a glance what is on offer on a weekly basis. For example, depending on the season, you might have the option of ordering a box which contains carrots, onions, lettuce, beetroot, apples, watercress and green cabbage.

However, if this combination was not to your taste, you have the option of ordering your own combination of fruits and vegetables from the general menu. What's more, the suppliers have now added many more organic products to their range; so it is possible to order the likes of organic free-range eggs, nuts and seeds, apple juice, canned tomatoes, dried fruits, pasta, bread, sauces, soups, and even non-toxic house cleaning products, which helps to reduce the environmental toxins in your home which may affect asthma and skin allergies.

It really is like having access to your own organic super-market and it can be fun to sit down with your child and go through some of the ordering options together, which is a great way to foster their appreciation of organic food.

If you want to look into it further I suggest you carry out an online search for local organic fruit and vegetable box schemes operating in your area. Some of the growers have open market gardens and cafe's that you can visit.

What About Growing Your Own?

Allotments are fun as well as being hard work. Even if you have no garden space, it is still possible to grow some organic produce in plant-pots or in window boxes. I know some people who grow organic carrots in deep-filled tubs which are kept on the patio. It is also a good idea to plant leafy crops such as little gem lettuce, spinach or corn salad (sometimes referred to as lamb's lettuce) as then you can be assured they won't have been grown using chemicals, if you use organic compost and no chemical slug pellets or sprays yourself.

These can provide a steady supply of greens for most of the year in places in temperate regions; or if you are lucky enough to live in warmer climes, you can grow fruits and vegetables all-year round outdoors. This is also a great way to save money as well as provide yourself and your children with chemical-free produce.

Sprouting

Another option you have is to try sprouting nuts, seeds, pulses and grains. For example, you can sprout the South American grain, Quinoa, and add it to salads all-year round. You can do the same with pulses such as chick-peas, aduki and mung beans. Even nuts such as almonds can be sprouted in this way. Some of the easiest and quickest sprouts to grow are broccoli and alfalfa, which may be ready in a few days.

In addition to being organically-grown, these sprouts are an excellent source of enzymes and nutrients for your child. They also contain a wide range of phytochemicals that offer protection against pollution and disease.

The enzymes in sprouts help to make them easily digestible and some nutritional experts, such as Dr Brian Clement, the Director of the Hippocrates Health Institute in Florida, believe that they have a part to play in disease prevention and recovery from illness. Two of the healthiest to grow are snow pea and sunflower sprouts. These are high in chlorophyll, which is thought to be very health-promoting. Sunflower sprouts are a great addition to sandwiches and salads. Kids like them for their nutty flavor.

How to Grow Sprouts

Before the nuts or seeds can sprout successfully, they must be soaked in water for a given time, and this will vary according to the seeds being sprouted. Generally speaking, the larger the seed, the longer the soaking time. For example, sunflower seeds need to be soaked for around 6 hours, whilst alfalfa seeds require five hours; pulses such as aduki beans and chick-peas need to be soaked for 12 hours.

At the end of this period simply drain and rinse the seeds and place them in a sprouting jar or if you wish to sprout more than one type of seed at the same time, purchase a sprouting unit which is made up of three, four or five trays stacked on top of each other.

Evenly distribute the seeds on each tray and water regularly. The water drains through each tray and collects in a reservoir at the bottom. This is simply emptied when full.

It's a great idea to get the kids involved as they love this kind of thing.

For more information on sprouting I suggest that you purchase the book, 'The Sprouter's Handbook', by Edward Cairney (Argyll Publishing). It is a wonderful easy-to-read reference guide to sprouting.

Wild Harvest

If you have access to the countryside it is worthwhile doing some research into which wild plants may be available to harvest. For instance, it is often possible to harvest edible wild berries that have not been sprayed (though be aware that hedgerows near farms may have been contaminated by the farmer spraying nearby fields). Blackberries and elderberries are rich in vitamin C and bioflavanoids and can be used fresh or made into healthy jams or drinks. Depending on where in the world you live, you can often find wild garlic growing in the woods and there is usually a number of wild herbs such as edible chick-weed, which tastes remarkably like lettuce (be sure you don't eat the non-edible version though as there are two types) and wild fennel..

When collecting wild plants or berries, it is a good idea to select produce that is not growing near busy roads where they are exposed to exhaust fumes. It's also not a good idea to harvest plants growing on the edge of farmer's fields where chemical sprays are being used, as these may have contaminated the wild plants or fruits that you are collecting.

Be very careful when collecting wild fungi. Some are poisonous and I was just reading in a national newspaper of one fatality involving an unfortunate lady who collected and consumed death cap mushrooms in the English countryside. In fact, even experienced wild mushroom collectors can sometimes be poisoned as a result of misidentification. So, my advice is: if you are going to collect wild fungi, get expert guidance.

If you would like to learn more on the subject of harvesting wild edible foods from the countryside, a good guide book is Richard Mabey's 'Food for Free' (Collins). A good reference book will also help to ensure that you select only safe, edible wild foods.

10

Healthy Meal Ideas

Salads!

Fair enough, when we think of children and salads, the words chalk and cheese tend to come to mind. However, if your child is salad phobic, it's worth trying them out with a few of the following ideas. The secret is to be as adventurous as possible. Basically we need to shatter the myth that salads have to be based upon boring lettuce and tomatoes:

Super Salad

The good thing about this salad is that there aren't any rules (except to use natural healthy ingredients of course!)

Preparation:

Using a large salad bowl, simply chop up any of your child's favourite vegetables, fruits, etc, and throw them into the mix. The following list of ingredients should mean that you are never short of ideas:

Apples
Alfalfa sprouts
Asparagus
Beans – green (runner beans or French beans)
Broad beans
Bean sprouts – these are packed with vitamins
Beetroot (either raw or cooked)
Broccoli
Cabbage (red or white, or make into coleslaw)
Carrots (grated or chopped)

Cauliflower

Celery

Chick peas (rich in protein)

Cucumber

Dates

Chicory

Zucchini (courgettes)

Lentils

Lettuce

Mushrooms

Mustard and cress

Onions

Peas

Peppers

Potatoes (cooked)

Pumpkin seeds

Raisins

Spinach

Sunflower seeds

Tomatoes

Watercress

Additional ingredients

Once you have your basic mixture, you might like to make your salad even more child-friendly by adding one or two of the following ingredients:

- Cheese (hard or soft, e.g. cottage cheese)

- Eggs – hard boiled (preferably organic/free-range)

- Fish – such as tuna, wild salmon or sardines

- Meat – white meats such as chicken are best

- Nuts – providing your child isn't allergic to them, try adding peanuts, cashews or almonds (Warning! These need to be ground up for small children to avoid choking.)

- Whole meal pasta – quick and easy to cook; try adding it to salads as a quick source of lasting energy

- Whole grains – cooked brown rice, couscous, quinoa

- Hummus – a savoury spread made from chick-peas, sesame seeds, lemon juice and vegetable oil – it's a very good source of protein and the sesame seeds in hummus are a good source of calcium too

These foods, when added to your salads, not only help to make them more interesting, but also provide a source of carbohydrates (pasta and whole grains), protein (fish, nuts, hummus, eggs, cheese, meats), vitamins and minerals (all of the above) and healthy fats (fish, nuts and hummus).

Salad dressings
Good salad dressings can make all the difference to a salad. You can either make your own, or you can buy some really good healthy ones from your local health food shop or super-market. Choose dressings that are made from natural ingre-dients and beware of added sugar and artificial sweeteners. Natural ingredients include the likes of cider vinegar (better for us than malt or spirit vinegar which can irritate the gut lining), honey or date syrup (instead of sugar), herbs and olive oil. There are also a good choice of natural mayonnaise dressings made from ingredients such as cider vinegar, lemon juice and free-range eggs. Just experiment and see what your child likes best.

Home-made Coleslaw
1/4 white cabbage, finely shredded
1 or 2 carrots finely grated
1 deseeded chopped red pepper
1 tbsp olive oil
1 tbsp natural mayonnaise
black pepper to taste

Preparation:
Place the vegetables in a bowl. Whisk together the oil and mayonnaise with a fork. Add some black pepper to taste. Pour the mixture over the vegetables and mix well. Serves 1-2.

Grated Carrots and Celeriac with Raisins or Dates
½ a celeriac peeled and grated
2 medium size carrots, grated
a handful of dates or raisins
1 tbsp natural mayonnaise or French dressing

Preparation:
Grate the celeriac and carrots and place in a bowl along with the raisins or dates. Pour the dressing over the mixture and mix well. Serve with whole wheat or whole rye bread, spread with a little butter or healthy margarine made from cold-pressed oils. Serves 1-2.

Brown Rice Salad
150g cooked brown rice
chopped red or yellow peppers
broad beans or peas
cider vinegar and oil dressing - 1 part vinegar to 2 parts oil
small bunch of watercress
Finely sliced raw red onion
handful of roasted peanuts

1 tbsp of raisins

Preparation:
Empty the cooked rice into a mixing bowl. Add the vegetables and roasted peanuts. Garnish with the watercress, add the vinegar and oil dressing to taste and mix well. Serves 2-3

Finger Salad
1 yellow pepper sliced
¼ raw cauliflower cut into bite-size pieces
1 medium carrot cut into sticks
1 stick of celery cut into sticks.
spring onions
cherry tomatoes

Preparation:
Serve the prepared vegetables with a favorite healthy dip (e.g. mint and yoghurt) or hummus, and include some rye crisp-bread spread with a little butter or healthy margarine. Serves 1-2.

Couscous Fruity Salad
100g (3½ oz) couscous
2 tbsp cooked peas
175ml boiling water/vegetable stock
chopped dried apricots
chopped cherry tomatoes
2 tbsp raisins or sultanas
1 tsp of allspice
1 tbsp of olive oil

Preparation:
This dish is quick and easy to prepare. Simply put the couscous in a bowl. Dissolve a vegetable stock in the boiling

water and add the stock to the couscous, then leave for around 5 minutes until the liquid is absorbed. Add the chopped fruit, vegetables, allspice and olive oil and mix well until fluffy. Serves 1-2.

Avocado, Tomato, Ice-Burg Lettuce and Prawn Salad
½ small tub of Icelandic prawns
4 tomatoes – sliced
1 cup of chopped iceberg lettuce
1 ripe avocado, stoned, peeled and sliced
2 tbsp of mayonnaise
1 tsp of cayenne pepper

Preparation:
Place the lettuce on a serving plate; add a layer of sliced tomatoes and sliced avocadoes. Mix the prawns with the mayonnaise and empty the mixture onto the middle of the plate. Sprinkle with the cayenne pepper and serve with slices of whole wheat bread or toast thinly spread with a little butter or healthy margarine. Serves 1-2.

Pasta Salad
150g whole wheat pasta
small can of sweet corn, drained and rinsed
1 medium zucchini (courgette) cut into small strips
2 spring onions, finely chopped
1 red and 1 yellow pepper, deseeded and finely sliced
80g of canned tuna

Preparation:
Bring a medium-sized pan of water to the boil, add the pasta and cook until just cooked (al dente).Drain and refresh in cold water. Drain and place in a salad bowl. Add the vegetables and tuna to the pasta; mix well and serve. Serves 1-2.

Rice and Baked Beans Salad

½ can of healthy baked beans
100g of whole-grain basmati rice
tomato sauce
chopped cherry tomatoes
1 grated carrot
1 red onion finely sliced
a handful of pine-nuts

Preparation:
Place the rice in a medium-sized pan of water. Bring to the boil, then simmer for 20 minutes. Drain the rice and allow to cool. Add the vegetables, pine-nuts and baked beans; mix well and serve.

Caesar Salad

1 cup shredded iceberg lettuce
1 medium grated carrot
chopped hard-boiled egg (preferably free-range)
25g Parmesan cheese
croutons (preferably whole meal)
French dressing (olive or walnut oil, wine vinegar, mustard)

Preparation:
Place the ingredients in a salad bowl, mix well and sprinkle with grated parmesan cheese. Serve with whole wheat or rye bread. Serves 1.

Cauliflower, Carrot, Beetroot and Chicken Salad

¼ raw cauliflower cut into bite size pieces
Handful of sunflower seeds
1 carrot, grated
Croutons (preferably whole meal)
favorite salad dressing

1 beetroot, grated
200g bite-sized pieces of cooked chicken*

Preparation:
Simply place the salad ingredients in a salad bowl; add the sunflower seeds, croutons, pieces of chicken and salad dressing; mix well and serve. Serves 1-2.

*Cut the chicken into very small pieces for small children to avoid danger of choking.

Cooked Meals

'Souper' kids

Soups can be a great way of getting your children to consume vegetables. They are both tasty and nutritious. If you have time to prepare your own soups all you need to do is stick to the basic formula which comprises your choice of vegetables, water and stock. Using this formula all you have to do is add your favorite additional ingredients, such as chicken, whole wheat pasta, herbs, noodles, croutons and cereals (e.g. barley and oats); and as a special treat, try adding a little fresh cream. Sometimes, even children who hate vegetables will happily consume soup, which is a good way of incorporating them into the diet.

The perfect complement to soup is crusty whole wheat or whole rye bread spread with a little butter or healthy margarine – delicious!

The following recipe is a typical example of a quickly prepared soup:

Lentil Soup
1 carrot finely chopped
1 stick of celery, finely chopped
1 onion, finely chopped

220g of pre-cooked red lentils
juice of a lemon
4 tbsp bio-yoghurt
1 tbsp olive oil
black pepper to taste
850mls of vegetable stock

Preparation:
Using a large saucepan gently sauté the onion with the olive oil. Add the vegetables and stock and briefly bring to the boil; then simmer for around 15-20 minutes. Add the lentils, pepper and lemon juice and simmer for another 5 minutes. Pour into serving bowls and add 1 tablespoon of bio-yoghurt if desired. Serve with whole wheat bread. Approximately 5 servings.

Shop bought soups

If you haven't the time to make your own soups, then don't worry, because there are lots of healthy versions available in cartons from health food shops and supermarkets. These come in a variety of flavors, including carrot and coriander, creamy tomato, pea, minestrone and tomato and lentil. Look out for the ones that are made from natural healthy ingredients, and avoid the one's that contain ingredients such as sugar and white flour; especially the supermarket's own brands. One thing I have noted is that supermarkets sometimes stock the healthiest brands, then after assessing their popularity, they will discard the original brand and replace this with their own version using inferior ingredients and slipping in a few of those additives we're trying to avoid.

Pizza

Let's face it, kids love pizzas! The trouble is that the combination of flour and cheese is not such a healthy one. Having said this, we have to be realistic because most children are going to want pizzas, at least occasionally. So, what's the answer?

Well, the best answer that I can think of is to make your own. It's fun to make pizza dough together (you can use a rice based gluten free flour and it won't taste any different from regular pizza). But if you're short of time, you can still make home made pizzas with great healthy toppings, using a ready-made whole wheat base. Just spread the base with canned chopped tomatoes, cheese and your child's favorite toppings such as pineapple and mushrooms. Place in the oven and cook until golden brown, and hey presto! You've got a delicious home-made pizza in minutes.

Incidentally, for those parents who have a child who is sensitive to wheat or gluten, you can now purchase gluten-free pizza bases, so they don't need to miss out on this occasional treat. In fact, as mentioned earlier in this book, some pizza chains are happy for you to bring in your own base and they will add your choice of toppings. This is a good option for all but the severely gluten sensitive child, since there is a danger of cross-contamination from the other flour being used.

Tuna Pasta
This is another quick meal which should appeal to busy parents.

225g of whole wheat pasta
1 large onion, thinly sliced
15g (1/2 oz) of olive oil
½ tsp of mixed herbs
1 tbsp of tomato puree
1 tin (440g) tomatoes
1 can (200g) of tuna fish
black pepper to taste.

Preparation:
Boil the pasta in plenty of unsalted water for approximately 10 minutes, until slightly tender. In the meantime, gently sauté

the onion in the oil for five minutes; then add all of the other ingredients. If desired, you can add peas, sweet corn or sliced mushrooms. Serves 4.

Fish Cakes

Fish cakes, like fish fingers, are often popular with children. They are a good source of protein and healthy fats. This home-made version uses healthy ingredients; however, it is possible to purchase some shop-bought versions which don't contain additives. Gluten-free versions for children on a wheat-free or gluten-free diet are also becoming available.

225g potatoes
225g of white fish
15g butter or healthy margarine
1 small onion, finely chopped
1 egg, beaten
2 tsp of tomato puree
50g whole meal breadcrumbs
1 lemon
15g parsley
¼ tsp of black pepper

Preparation:
Wash and cut the potato into cubes. Cook in a small amount of boiling water. Cut the fish into small pieces and add to the pan of boiling potatoes. Cook for a further 10 minutes; then simmer for 5 minutes. Meanwhile, mix half the beaten egg, tomato puree, onion, salt and pepper. Drain the fish and potatoes and remove any bones from the fish. Mash the potatoes with the butter or margarine. Add the fish and egg mixture to the potatoes and mix well.

Shape into fish cakes, adding some of the breadcrumbs; then dip in remaining egg in order to make the breadcrumbs adhere. Lightly fry the fishcakes in a little oil for a few minutes, turning once. Alternatively, grill or bake in the oven for a few minutes. Serves 4.

Sweet Potato Mash
This is a nice change from ordinary potatoes and a good source of nutrients. Kids love the sweet creamy taste.

4 medium-sized sweet potatoes
1-2 tsp of olive or cold-pressed sunflower oil

Preparation:
Peel then cut the sweet potatoes into quarters. Put about 5cm (2in) of water in a saucepan and bring to the boil. Add the sweet potatoes and bring back to the boil. Simmer for a further 15-20 minutes until softened. Drain and return them to the saucepan. Now add the oil and mash until smooth and creamy. Serve with other vegetables and healthy baked beans if desired. Serves 3-4.

Steam-Fried Vegetables
This is a much healthier alternative to stir-frying vegetables and is lower in calories too!

your choice of chopped vegetables –
spring onions
mushrooms
sugar snap peas
finely sliced julienne carrots
sliced red pepper
chopped celery
zucchini
fresh peas

Preparation:

Add a small amount of olive oil to a pan or wok and heat gently for 1 minute. Then add a water-based sauce such as tamari or soy sauce and add the vegetables. Cover with a lid and cook. This process steams the food whilst at the same time imparting the full flavor of the oil and sauce to the food. This method ensures that you avoid the production of oxidants and also a toxic substance called acrylamide, which is produced when food is burnt.

As with a large mixed salad, you can be as adventurous as you like with your choice of ingredients. Vegetables should represent the bulk of the ingredients; however, you can add all sorts of other ingredients, such as tuna, pine-nuts, sultanas, bean sprouts, whole wheat pasta or chicken. Just experiment and see what your child likes best. You can also serve this dish with whole grain rice or basmati rice.

Healthy Oven Chips

This version is both quick to prepare and healthier because olive oil is used instead of the other less stable polyunsaturated oils, which are damaged by heat and produce unhealthy fats:

2 tbsp of extra virgin olive oil
2 large potatoes, peeled and chopped into chips (fries)
pinch of paprika (optional)

Preparation:

Pre-heat the oven to 220 degrees C/435 degrees F. Toss the chips in the oil and place in a lightly oiled baking tray. Sprinkle lightly with paprika, if desired. Cook for approximately 20-25 minutes, turning the chips once, until crispy. Serve with healthy baked beans and salad of your choice. Makes 2-3 servings.

Cheesy Parsnip and Potato Mash
2 large potatoes, peeled and cut into chunks
1 tbsp of butter/healthy margarine
2 tbsp of milk or soya milk
black pepper to taste
2 tbsp of grated parmesan cheese

Preparation:
Put 2 inches of water in a medium-sized pan and bring to the boil. Add the parsnips and potatoes. Reduce the heat and cook for a further 15 minutes until soft. Drain and add the butter, milk and black pepper and mash until a creamy texture is achieved. Serve and sprinkle with the parmesan cheese. It is excellent with cooked vegetables, peas, or runner beans. Serves 2-3.

Spanish Omelet
Spanish omelets are another good way of craftily increasing your child's vegetable intake.

1 cup of grated carrot
1 large onion thinly sliced
1 cup of runner beans
1 potato, sliced into discs and boiled
1 small tin of tomatoes
3 eggs
1 tbsp of vegetable oil

Preparation:
Using a frying pan (skillet), cook the onions. Add the tomatoes to the onions, add the runner beans and grated carrot and cook for a further 2 minutes. Meanwhile, beat the eggs and add seasoning if desired.

Stir the contents of the pan and move to one side before

adding the rest of the oil. Cook the potatoes lightly Then spread the vegetables evenly inside the pan and add the egg mixture. Stir the vegetable and egg mixture until the underneath begins to set. Turn over once and heat until just set. Remove from pan, cut into slices and serve. Serves 2.

Mixed Vegetable and Chick Pea Curry

If your child likes curries or can develop a taste for them, this is a good way of increasing their intake of healthy vegetables. Chick peas are an excellent source of protein and also magnesium, a mineral which is often lacking in junk food diets.

1 onion, finely chopped
1 tbsp tomato puree
2 zucchini (courgettes) diced
1 medium cauliflower – cut into pieces
1 medium carrot, diced
1 small pot of bio-yoghurt or 100ml coconut milk
½ can (200g) of ready-cooked chick peas
300 ml water or vegetable stock
1 tbsp olive oil
2 tbsp of mild vegetable curry

Preparation:
Sauté the onion in a frying pan with the oil until softened. Add the other vegetables and cook for another 3 minutes. Add the chick peas, tomato puree, curry paste and vegetable stock or water. Simmer for 20 minutes. Turn off the heat and allow to cool down before adding the yoghurt or coconut milk. Serve with whole grain rice or quinoa. Makes 2-3 servings.

Roasted Vegetables

This dish is quick and easy to prepare and is often liked by kids who love the sweet-tasting vegetables.

1 medium carrot
1 medium beetroot
½ small celeriac
1 medium parsnip
1 tsp of dried mixed herbs
2-3 tbsp olive oil
½ medium sweet potato
1 red or yellow pepper

Preparation:
Cut the beetroot, carrot, sweet potato and parsnip into the size of thick chips. Cut the sweet potato and parsnip into slightly larger chips to allow for shrinkage. Wash, deseed the pepper and cut into strips about 1cm (1/2 inch wide). Mix the dried herbs with the oil. Brush some of the oil onto a baking tray and heat in the oven for 3 minutes. Place the vegetables in the tin and brush with the oil. Place the tray back in the oven and bake for approximately 20-30 minutes until the vegetables are tender. Remove from the oven and remove any excess oil with a kitchen towel.

Can be eaten on its own or accompanied with a baked ready-made veggie sausage (healthy versions are available from health food shops and some supermarkets). Alternatively, you can add a piece of grilled fish or home-made fish-cake. Serves 2.

Nut Slice
1 large red onion, grated
100g (4oz) mushrooms
25g (1oz) toasted whole wheat breadcrumbs
1 tsp of dried mixed herbs
2 eggs
25g (1oz) soy flour
100g (4oz) mixed ground nuts

45g (1 ½ oz) sunflower seeds
25g (1oz) olive oil or cold pressed sunflower oil
150ml of stock
45g (1 ½ oz) sesame seeds

Preparation:
Pre-heat the oven to 375 degrees F/190 degrees C. Place the grated onion into a mixing bowl and add the nuts, seeds, flour, herbs, oil and salt. Beat the eggs and add them to the mixture. Chop the mushrooms and add. Empty the mixture into a suitable pie dish, sprinkle with breadcrumbs. Pour over the stock and bake for approximately 25-30 minutes. Serve either as a hot or cold dish with a green salad. Serves 3-4.

Turkey Bolognaise
This is a variation of regular bolognaise, substituting low fat turkey mince for beef mince, and whole wheat spaghetti instead of white; as these ingredients represent a healthier option.

1 red or yellow pepper, deseeded and sliced
1 large onion, sliced
225g (½ pound lean turkey mince)
3 tbsp tomato puree
400g (14oz) tinned, chopped tomatoes
1 tbsp of olive oil
1 tbsp dried mixed herbs
pinch of black pepper
Whole wheat spaghetti

Preparation:
Pour the oil into a frying pan or skillet, and sauté the onions and peppers for 2-3 minutes until tender. Add the chopped tomatoes, tomato paste, black pepper and herbs, whilst stirring to mix well. Cover then simmer for 8-10 minutes.

Cook the spaghetti in water until tender. Serve the spaghetti with the sauce and lightly sprinkle with Parmesan cheese if desired. Serves 2-3.

Healthy Fast Food Meals for Busy Parents

- Baked potato with a little butter or healthy margarine, filled with cottage cheese, healthy canned baked beans (e.g. Whole Earth) or hummus. Serve with a side salad.

- Potato and carrot mash. Boil and mash the vegetables with 1 tbsp of butter or healthy margarine; add a little salt and black pepper. Serve with healthy canned baked beans.

- Grilled or lightly fried veggie burger or bean burger (available from health food shops and supermarkets). Serve in a whole wheat roll or with whole meal rye bread with added lettuce and tomato.

- Whole wheat pitta bread lightly toasted and filled with a chopped boiled egg or low-fat cheese and sweet corn

- Home-made spicy beans on toast. Add some mild curry powder and sultanas to a can of healthy canned baked beans. Heat and eat on whole wheat toast or rye crisp bread.

- Baked potato and pizza topping. Bake the potato in the oven and add chopped mushrooms, red or yellow peppers and a natural tomato sauce. Grate some cheese as a topping; or you can use one of the excellent soy alternative cheeses if you prefer a healthier option.

- Yoghurt with potatoes and canned chick peas (preferably unsalted). Boil the potatoes until tender and cut them into small pieces. Place them in a bowl and add rinsed canned chick peas; stir in one pot of natural bio-yoghurt and add some black pepper, a pinch of sea-salt and a pinch of chilli powder.

- Spicy rice and lentils. Cook whole grain rice in water. When cooked mix with canned or home-cooked lentils. Heat 1 tbsp of olive oil in a pan and stir in some curry powder and a pinch of sea-salt. Add the curry sauce to the rice and lentil mixture and stir well. Serve with grilled chicken pieces, or use smoked tofu pieces as a vegetarian alternative.

- Sweet potato and chicken breast. Cook the sweet potatoes in water until tender and serve with skinless chicken breast and salad or vegetables.

- Mediterranean rice dish. Cook enough whole grain rice for two. Add some organic Mediterranean tomato sauce and mix well. Add chopped tomatoes, canned unsweetened sweet corn and canned chick peas. Serve with a salad or extra vegetables.

- Couscous or quinoa served with chopped bell peppers, onions, tomatoes and canned chick peas or healthy baked beans. Serve with canned wild salmon or tuna.

- Corn chips served with carrot, celery, red, yellow or red peppers and cucumber. Use a healthy salsa dip or hummus for dipping

- Healthy baked beans on whole wheat or rye toast served with a salad (you can include the likes of baby spinach, cherry tomatoes, iceberg lettuce, raw cauliflower, spring onions, whole wheat croutons, grated carrot and radishes)

Healthy Snacks

It is easy to equate snacks with unhealthy choices; however, this doesn't have to be the case, since there are lots of healthy options to present to your children. Hopefully the following suggestions will help to get you on the right track:

- Fresh fruit – choose apples, pears, kiwi-fruit, strawberries, pineapple, oranges, peaches, grapes, melon, bananas or whatever is in season. Melons are best eaten on their own away from other fruits. This is due to the fact that they are digested very quickly and if mixed with other fruits that digest at a slower rate, may result in indigestion and gas. The same is true of grapes.

- Dried fruit (in moderation) – Choose unsulfured and preservative-free raisins, sultanas, apricots, dates, figs and currents.

- Popcorn – making home-made popcorn is a fun activity and it's so easy to make and much healthier than the commercial stuff. Cook the corn in a frying pan or skillet in a little olive oil and a teaspoonful of fructose (fruit sugar) or honey.

- Crudités –raw vegetables such as carrot, zucchini (courgette), celery, cucumber, mushroom and cucumber cut into bite-size pieces. They are delicious with a natural dip such as salsa, hummus or yoghurt dressing.

- Oatcakes – can be eaten with a little butter or healthy margarine; or try a healthy vegetarian savory spread like mushroom or lentil pate

- You can purchase healthy packet snacks from health food shops and some supermarkets with health food shelves.

The good ones are free from chemical additives (like monosodium glutamate) and low in salt. Lots of tasty treats are becoming widely available.

- Rice cakes – spread with unsweetened jam (sweetened with concentrated fruit juice instead of sugar; but avoid artificial sweeteners like the plague!)

- Rice cakes, spread with hummus and topped with a slice of tomato, or spread with peanut butter, almond butter or mixed nut butter (available from health food shops). The raw nut butter versions (not roasted) are the healthiest since the healthy fats in them have not been subjected to heat.

- Corn cakes – a substitute for rice cakes if preferred

- Home-made cakes made from whole wheat or whole rye flour and sweetened with honey, date syrup or molasses. Wheat and Gluten-free cakes can be made using appropriate specialized flours now available from many supermarkets and health food stores. Opt for gluten-free flour that has not been refined whenever possible.

- Nuts and raisins – always a good energy sustaining snack. N.B. exercise caution when feeding very young children nuts and seeds due to potential choking hazard.

- Seeds – children can develop a taste for the likes of sunflower, pumpkin and shelled hemp seeds. These seeds are packed with healthy Omega 3 and Omega 6 fats which are good for the immune system, circulation and for brain function.

- Soy nuts – these are made from roasted soy beans and are a good source of protein

Healthy Desserts

Let's face it, most children love sweet stuff! So it is important to present them with healthier options whenever possible. The following ideas should help to get you started:

Ice-cream

This doesn't have to be unhealthy as long as your child doesn't eat too much of it. Look out for ice-cream that has been made from only natural ingredients and sweetened with healthier ingredients such as honey. There are some delicious versions available from health food shops and some supermarkets these days. For children unable to tolerate cow's milk products, you can purchase ice-cream made from goat's milk, which is sometimes better tolerated. Also, look out for alternatives such as rice or soy ice-cream, as these can be a healthier alternative to the dairy version.

Beware of those packed with sugar though. It is now possible to purchase ice-cream that is made from creamed nuts (such as cashew), a small amount of honey and natural flavorings such as vanilla and cocoa. These are very pure and taste delicious. They also have the advantage of being much healthier than ice-cream that is made from cow's milk.

Soy desserts

There are now some very nice soy desserts to choose from. They come in a variety of flavors, such as chocolate, strawberry, carob and vanilla. Try to opt for brands that are made from organic soy beans, as these will also be GMO free.

Carob

Carob comes from the carob bean. The pods have a pleasant sweet taste and when ground into powder, they are used to make chocolate-like confectionary. Some of the carob bars that you can buy are very tasty and serve as a good alternative to chocolate as they are caffeine-free.

Real custard

Packets of natural custard powder are available from most health food shops. They are easy to make, so give them a try. You can serve them with fruits such as apricots and chopped bananas which will increase your child's fruit intake.

Sorbets

Most commercially produced sorbets are packed with white sugar, so beware! It is possible to buy healthier versions in some health food shops; or you can make your own using natural unsweetened fruit juices, or squeezed lemon juice and a little natural sweetener such as honey. Use a suitable freezable container, add the mixture and simply freeze.

Ice-lollipops

Simply pour the juice of your choice into a lollipop mould and place in the freezer. There are plenty of unsweetened juices to choose from, including pineapple, apple, orange and the more exotic juices such as kiwi and mango. I would always advise parents to opt for organic juices wherever possible.

Fresh fruit and bio-yoghurt

The slightly sour flavor of natural bio-yoghurt makes a good combination with sweet succulent fruits such as kiwi, grapes, melon, apple and pear. These yoghurts also contain live healthy bacteria which are good for the health of the digestive system.

Drinks

The secret behind weaning your child off those sugar and additive-packed fizzy drinks is to introduce them to the following alternatives:

- Fruit juice – dilute with an equal amount of pure water. Children often like apple, pear, grape and orange; however, there are now an increasing number of exotic juices becoming popular; such as pomegranate and mango.

- Smoothies – these are made by liquidizing the likes of soy, oat milk, almond milk or bio-yoghurt with honey, bananas, strawberries, pears, kiwi fruits and blueberries. Great as an energy-booster between meals, or at breakfast time. Also, a good source of nutrients and antioxidants.

- Raw juices – if you own a juice extractor, you can make your children some interesting juice combinations, such as apple, celery and carrot. These are very detoxifying and great for boosting your child's immune system.

- Herb teas – a great alternative to ordinary tea which contains stimulants. There are some interesting flavors to choose from, including, mint, spearmint, fennel and lime blossom. Sweeten with a little honey (avoid giving honey to children under one year old as their digestive systems are not ready to digest it at this stage).

- Coffee substitutes – these are caffeine-free and, unlike ordinary coffee, will not interfere with your child's blood sugar levels. Choose the likes of chicory and grain-based coffee substitutes which are available from health food shops and some supermarkets.

- Home-made lemonade – this is a great alternative to the additive and sugar packed commercial variety. Simply pour the juice of one lemon, 50ml of sparkling spring water and 3 or 4 tbsp of fruit concentrate (e.g. apple or pear) into a liquidizer and liquidize. Pour into a jug and serve.

Healthy Breakfasts

The following healthy breakfasts will help to sustain your child's energy levels throughout the first part of the day. In so doing, he/she will be able to concentrate better and will be less prone to mood swings:

- Banana milkshake made in a blender using one glass of semi-skimmed milk, or soy milk. Add one chopped banana and liquidize until smooth and frothy. For those children who are allergic to soy or cow's milk try almond or oat milk as an alternative.

- One or two slices of whole wheat or rye toast spread with a little butter or healthy margarine and unsweetened jam; e.g. bilberry or blackcurrant sweetened with concentrated apple juice. Children on a gluten-free diet can have toasted gluten-free bread. The healthy versions made with whole grain flour (e.g. brown rice flour instead of white) are best.

- Bio-yoghurt with a handful of raisins or sultanas; sprinkle with some sesame seeds or hulled hempseeds if desired

- Toasted whole wheat pitta bread filled with a little honey or peanut, almond, or other nut butter

- Swiss style muesli with semi-skimmed milk, soy, almond or rice milk Add fresh fruit for extra fiber and nutrients.

- Unsweetened canned fresh fruit served with natural bio-yoghurt. Choose from pear slices, pineapple, peaches or mixed fruit cocktail.

- Whole wheat toast spread with a little butter or healthy margarine and some nut or seed butter. Choose from the likes of peanut, almond, pumpkin or sunflower.

- Whole wheat muffin spread with a little butter and low-fat cream cheese or hummus

- Homemade muesli – simply mix your own blend of grains in flake form and add the likes of nuts, seeds, raisins, dates or sultanas. Flaked grains are available from health food shops and include buckwheat, rice, wheat, rye, quinoa and oats. For those children on a wheat or gluten-free diet, parents can easily make a specialized muesli using grains that they can eat.

- Rye crisp bread or oatcakes spread with a little butter or healthy margarine and hummus or tahini (sesame seed spread) – a good source of healthy fats, protein and calcium

- If you own a sandwich maker you can use whole wheat or rye bread to make healthy toasties. Choose from a variety of fillings; including banana and nut butter, unsweetened jam, or honey.

- No cook quick porridge – Before retiring for bed, pour some oat flakes into a breakfast bowl and cover with some semi-skimmed milk , soy or rice milk. Add a little honey or dried fruit. Cover and place in the fridge. In the morning remove from fridge and serve as ready-made cold porridge.

Packed Lunches

The challenge with packed lunches is how to make them interesting as well as balanced and healthy. You are also going to be competing with the 'junk' food contents of other kid's packed lunches; so it is important to compromise and allow the odd treat, such as a small bar of chocolate. This can be of the best quality, such as those made with dark chocolate and devoid of unhealthy hydrogenated fats.

Here are some ideas:

- Whole wheat toasty filled with nut or seed butter

- Tuna mayonnaise sandwich with iceberg lettuce and sweet corn

- Corn chips – natural flavor is healthiest as they are less likely to contain additives. Include a small pot of healthy salsa dip if desired. Look for corn chips that are made from whole grain corn.

- Whole wheat or rye bread, egg, cress and mayonnaise sandwich, cut into wedge shapes

- Bio-yoghurt or soy yoghurt

- Packet of nuts, or seeds, with added dried fruit – not suitable for very young children due to danger of choking

- Small bar of good quality chocolate

- Carrot and celery sticks with slices of cucumber and favorite natural dip; e.g. hummus

- Cheese or soy cheese slice in a whole wheat roll and natural pickle

- Small mixed salad – include ingredients such as tomatoes, cooked wholegrain rice (flavored with tamari sauce), zucchini (courgettes), grated carrot, beetroot and baby spinach or iceberg lettuce). Include a small tub of your child's favorite dressing if desired.

- Fruit bar – made without added sugar. These come in a variety of flavors, including pineapple, dates, raisins, apricot, mango, coconut, apple and pear; or combinations of these.

- Whole wheat or rye chicken sandwich with pickle or chutney. It is advisable to avoid buying packaged chicken slices as these often contain the additive sodium nitrite – which forms carcinogenic substances known as nitrosamines. Better to use thinly sliced fresh chicken prepared at home.

- Small packet of raisins, apricots or sultanas (preferably organic)

- Piece of fruit or small bunch of grapes

- Vegetable crisps – a nice alternative to ordinary crisps. Some brands include sugar, so try to avoid those. They are available from supermarkets and most health food stores. Choose from beetroot, parsnip, carrot and sweet potato crisps.

- Potato crisps and other savory snacks. These don't need to be unhealthy as there are brands that use natural ingredients and are low in salt. Available from health food shops and some supermarkets.

- Soy dessert – these come in handy tubs and are available in a variety of flavors, including chocolate, vanilla and fruit flavors.

Striking a Good Balance

When preparing a packed lunch it is a good idea to attempt to strike a balance between the fruits and vegetable ingredients and the starchy and high protein foods. Try to include something from each category in your child's lunch-box. For example, if you include a chicken sandwich, this is high in starch (from the bread) and protein (from the chicken),

Be sure to include some vegetables in some form, or fruit. This creates a good balance between major food groups.

11

Veggie Kids!

There are an increasing number of children switching to vegetarianism these days. In some cases they just decide that they don't want to eat animals any more. This sometimes happens when a child discovers what is involved when animals are slaughtered for food. Some children are vegetarian on environmental grounds; some are vegetarian for religious reasons. Then there is the child who just doesn't like the taste of meat. For some reason they just don't like the flavor, or maybe the texture of meat.

More rarely, some children decide to become vegetarian because they are aware of the health benefits associated with living largely on fruits and vegetables. This can be when a teenager becomes fixated on a rigorous diet with a hint of self-denial. This latter example is usually the result of parental influence where one or both parents are vegetarians and attempt to impress upon their child the value of vegetarianism; or in some cases veganism.

Sometimes it is the case where a child or teenager wants to exert control and does this through what they agree and refuse to eat.

To be more specific, there are various types of vegetarians, which fall into the following categories:

Lacto-ovo-vegetarian: someone who eats eggs and dairy products.
Lacto-vegetarian: someone who eats dairy products, but no eggs.
Vegan: someone who eats no animal products at all, including no dairy products, and lives on pulses, grains, legumes,

nuts, seeds, fruits and vegetables.

Semi-vegetarian: do not eat meat, but will eat some animal produce in the form of eggs, dairy and often fish.

Now whilst I acknowledge that there are many adult and child vegetarians and vegans who are perfectly healthy, and indeed in some instances they can be healthier than their meat-eating counterparts; there are many vegetarians who have developed some very bad dietary habits indeed! Put simply:

There are lots of vegetarians and vegans out there who not only look ill; they are ill!

So, why is this happening? The answer is simple; in their efforts to avoid meat (or if vegan, all animal products), whether for health or moral reasons, they have substituted other foods that if eaten in excess are very unhealthy!

As a vegan, it is very easy to adhere to a diet that is too restricting, resulting in deficiencies of various nutrients, such as vitamin B12, iron and Vitamin D. All of which are more amply supplied when certain foods from animals are part of the diet.

To visualize how deficiencies and imbalances occur, it might be useful to analyze the following types of vegetarian diet. We will begin by outlining what might be a typical day's eating. Let's call this first example Child A:

Child A
Breakfast:
Muesli with cow's milk
Whole wheat toast and strawberry jam
Lunch:
Cheese sandwich
Shop-bought salad comprising: tomatoes, onions, red peppers, creamy pasta in mayonnaise, coleslaw

Dessert: yoghurt and fresh fruit

Evening meal:

Macaroni cheese (made with white pasta), steamed vegetables, baked beans

Dessert: apple crumble (made with white flour and white sugar) and organic ice-cream

Snacks during the day: nuts and raisins, whole meal biscuits, packet of crisps or corn chips

Now let's take a look at an average day's eating for Child B:

Child B

Breakfast:

Whole-wheat toast spread with a thin layer of butter or almond nut butter

Fresh fruit salad sprinkled with hulled hemp seeds and ground flaxseeds

Cup of herb or fruit tea sweetened with a little honey

Lunch:

Mixed vegetable and aduki bean soup served with crusty whole wheat or whole rye bread spread with a little butter or healthy margarine

Dessert: bio yoghurt flavored with blueberries; or use soy yoghurt.

Cup of tea with soy milk and sweetened with a little honey

Evening meal:

Brown rice risotto; comprising chopped mixed vegetables, whole grain brown rice, chopped hard boiled egg, flavored with a vegetable stock-cube and layered with a small amount of grated Parmesan cheese

Dessert: home-made lemon sorbet

Cup of peppermint tea sweetened with a little honey.

Snacks during the day: oat bar, small packet of apricots, nuts and raisins, chocolate bar, rice-cake spread with hummus

How They Compare

Child A

When we look carefully at what types of foods Child A consumes on an average day, we can see that he/she relies heavily on dairy produce. This is such a common occurrence when people switch from meat-eating to the lacto-vegetarian type of diet, or in this case a lacto-ovo vegetarian diet, since eggs are included.

The problem with eating too many dairy foods is:

- They are highly mucous-forming (which can lead to snuffles).

- They contain a high level of calcium compared to their magnesium content; which is fine for developing calves, but unsuitable for humans.

- They are high in saturated fats which are linked with an increase in heart disease and circulatory disorders in humans.

- They are one of the foods that adults and children are most likely to become intolerant or allergic to. The propensity of young children to develop lactose (milk sugar) intolerance or allergy increases when weaned onto cow's milk as babies. In such cases the infant may be reacting to any one of a number of milk proteins present in the milk; or they may lack the enzyme lactase, necessary for digesting the lactose.

Many naturopaths and nutritional practitioners have observed that lacto-vegetarian adults and children, who base their diets largely on dairy products, often have a rather pale or pasty complexion. This is due to the mucus-forming properties of the milk, cheese and flour products such as pasta, bread and spaghetti. It is the gluten content of wheat that makes them 'gluey' or glutinous. This is easily demonstrated if we add flour to water, which produces a paste-like substance – in fact it was used as wallpaper paste in the past.

In addition to the emphasis upon dairy products, this diet is also heavily weighted in favor of wheat products, especially pasta; which in this case happens to be the white refined version.

This is unhealthy for a number of reasons, namely:

- Eating a lot of wheat and wheat-based products may predispose an individual towards developing a wheat or gluten intolerance or allergy (see chapter 7, Allergic Kids!).

- Wheat contains a natural compound known as phytic acid, which is a chelator (binds with) of minerals such as calcium, magnesium and zinc. Therefore, a diet that is high in wheat may reduce availability of these minerals from the foods we eat.

- Most of the wheat in this diet is refined. Therefore, it is low in fiber and nutrients. Also, it is known that refined carbo-hydrates such as white flour and its products use up the body's own supply of nutrients in order to digest them; for example, B vitamins.

Acid/Alkaline Balance

Finally, most naturopaths and nutritional practitioners agree that in health the body needs to be slightly alkaline, with a blood pH of around 7.4. What happens when we eat too many acid-forming foods is that the pH changes, resulting in an over-acid system.

This in turn may weaken the immune system, which in turn can lead to a greater susceptibility to illness. The majority of foods in child A's diet are acid-forming. This is why it's important that fruits and vegetables are eaten in good quantities on a daily basis, since they are our greatest source of alkaline-forming minerals; for example, potassium and magnesium.

I always suggest that parents try to plan their child's diet around the 80:20 rule. That is, the diet should consist of around 80% vegetables with some fruits, and 20% acid-forming foods such as nuts, seeds, grains and pulses.

If your child is on a lacto-vegetarian diet, you would include cheese as an acid-forming food. Fish-eating vegetarians also need to bear in mind that fish is acid-forming, as are meats for non-vegans and non-vegetarians. Acid-forming foods need to be eaten in much smaller quantities compared to the alkaline-forming fruits and vegetables.

If you find it difficult to implement the 80:20 rule, then you might need to compromise by adjusting it to something like 60:40 to begin with; or even 50:50. You can then increase the alkaline-forming foods gradually over a period of time.

Conclusion

Child A's diet is typically associated with wheat based products, coupled with lots of dairy foods such as cheese, milk and yoghurt. The end result is an individual who is often mucous-congested, tired and prone to illness.

Child B's diet, despite the inclusion of some unhealthy foods, is undoubtedly more nutritionally balanced and nutrient-rich. It is a healthier vegetarian diet because:

- It includes mostly whole grains such as brown rice, whole wheat and whole rye.

- It is more alkaline than child B's diet since it includes more fruits and vegetables at each meal.

- It includes flax and hemp seeds which are rich in essential fatty acids; these are so important for good health and normal brain function – especially important for developing children.

- It is quite low in saturated fats.

- It provides a good range of vitamins, minerals and phyto-nutrients so essential in maintaining good health and resistance to disease.

- It provides a good supply of protein derived from nuts, seeds, whole grains and pulses.

- It is low in refined sugars.

- It provides enough vitamin B12 from eggs and dairy foods to meet daily requirements. The only reliable source of B12 is from animal sources.

- It includes some vitamin D from eggs and a little from the dairy products. This is especially important for children who live in regions where regular exposure to sunshine is limited since when the skin is exposed to the UVB rays in sunshine it can manufacture its own vitamin D; otherwise we rely almost entirely on dietary sources.

Conclusion

Child B's diet is much healthier overall and is likely to result in an alkaline system, stronger immune system and greater resistance to illness. Also, since most of the carbohydrates are of the whole grain variety, blood-sugar levels are likely to be fairly stable. If you remember, this is due to the fact that grains such as whole grain rice and whole meal bread are high in fiber, which results in slow conversion into glucose in the blood. This is also true when raw foods such as vegetables and fruits are eaten, since their high fiber content act like a 'brake' upon energy conversion in the body. The fact that there is a variety of grains in this diet instead of relying on wheat means that there will be less chance of developing wheat and/or gluten-intolerance.

Vegan Diets

Just as you might expect, bearing in mind how easy it is to fall into the poor vegetarian diet trap; there are plenty of unhealthy vegans out there who have followed suit. It's easy to see why when we take into account the fact that foods such as red meats are rich in iron, and vitamin B12, which is sometimes lacking in vegan diets, and is most abundant in meat, eggs and dairy products.

Also, in the light of current research, it is easy to overlook vitamin D. Recent studies have shown that this vitamin is commonly deficient, even in non-vegetarians.

When it comes to ensuring that your child has an adequate intake of iron, we must remember that the type of iron known as haem iron is derived from animal foods such as liver and red meats. This type of iron is well-absorbed by the body.

Iron from vegetable sources is known as non-haem iron. The absorption of this type of iron is much lower. That is not to say that this is going to be a major problem in vegan diets providing that the diet contains iron-rich plants such as broccoli, dark green leafy vegetables, pumpkin seeds, cooked beans, lentils and blackstrap molasses (this can be used in baking; for example it can be added to bread flour when baking bread; or to a cake mixture). Also, so called superfoods such as spirulina, a type of algae, are a good source of iron.

Iron absorption can be enhanced in the presence of vitamin C. So, if fruit that contains a good level of vitamin C, such as oranges or kiwi, are included in the same meal as a baked potato, cooked beans and broccoli, then the iron will be much better absorbed by the body.

What About Vitamin B12?

One of the biggest pit-falls associated with a vegan diet is not getting enough vitamin B12. This is not to be taken lightly, since a deficiency can lead to anemia and B12 neuropathy involving the degeneration of nerve fibers and in some cases irreversible nerve damage can occur. What it comes down to is that vegans should ensure that they are consuming B12 fortified foods on a daily basis. These include:

- Some fortified plant milks

- Fortified soy milk

- Some B12 fortified cereals

In addition to fortified foods, if you or your child is adhering to a vegan diet, then I would strongly recommend that you take a supplement that contains B12. I have contacted both UK based companies, Higher Nature and Biocare for advice on children and B12; they do offer supplements that contain this vitamin, which are as follows:

Biocare
Vitasorb – B12 in liquid form
Kids Complete – a multi vitamin/mineral capsule for slightly older children
Kids complex powder – for younger children when swallowing tablets or capsules might present a problem with choking
Higher Nature

Dinochews – chewable multi vitamin and mineral tablets for children

What About Vitamin D?

Recent research has indicated that vitamin D deficiency may be widespread, even amongst meat eaters. This is partly due to the fact that vitamin D is not plentiful in many everyday foods. Some foods such as eggs and fish contain this vitamin at a reasonable level; however, even eggs contain only around 20iu (international units) per egg. Therefore, in order to derive 400iu daily (a level thought by many scientists to be inadequate in the light of current research), you would need to consume 20 eggs. This would of course be highly undesirable as well as impracticable. Oily fish, such as salmon, does contain more significant amounts of vitamin D, with 4ozs providing approximately 400iu.

However, it is unlikely that your child will be eating the quantities required to off-set deficiencies and optimize the level required for good health. Other food sources include fortified foods, such as some margarine, soy milk and breakfast cereals. These are especially important for vegetarians and vegans, since apart from nettles and special mushrooms grown under ultra violet light, there is no vitamin D in plant foods.

Sunshine and Vitamin D

Vitamin D deficiency is also more likely if you live in a country where you get limited exposure to sunlight, as vitamin D is also manufactured by the skin when exposed to UV-B rays. However, it appears that we cannot necessarily rely upon sun exposure to provide us and our children with enough vitamin D either. Essentially, the closer one lives to the equator the more chance that you will be exposed to the all important UV-B rays. It is these rays that the body uses to manufacture vitamin D when skin is exposed.

Whilst UV-A solar radiation is present throughout a typical

sunny day, the amount of UV-B sunlight is only present on the hottest days and during the middle of the day. Also, the distance one lives from the equator determines the degree and length of UV-B exposure. In fact, some experts believe that if you live more than 30 degrees north or south of the equator, you may not be able to manufacture enough vitamin D from the sun on a year-round basis. This means getting the rest from foods and/or supplements. Of course, if you live in northern climates such as northern Europe or the UK (which begins at around 50 degrees latitude in the south of the UK), then supplementation, especially amongst vegetarians and vegans, is likely to be a necessity.

Symptoms of Vitamin D Deficiency

A deficiency of this vitamin results in a loss of calcium and phosphates in the stools, resulting in a fall in their blood level and subsequent poor bone formation. As a result, children can develop rickets, when the bones become soft and easily bent. A lack of this vitamin has also been linked with an increase in dental caries and poor immune function.

Recommended Dosage

Dr John Jacob Cannell, executive director of the USA based Vitamin D Council, states that healthy children under the age of one year old who have little UV-B exposure, should take 1,000iu of vitamin D3 Daily (D3 is the recommended version rather than another form of the vitamin known as vitamin D2). Over the age of one he recommends taking 1,000iu for every 25 pounds of body weight per day.

He further suggests that well adults and adolescents should take 5,000iu per day for two to three months, and then get a 25 (OH) D test (25 hydroxy) through their GP. Be sure to request this test as opposed to the 1.25-dihydroxy-vitamin D test that some doctors will order. Remember, these levels may vary according to your geographical location. Obviously, a child living in Miami will be better off regarding sunlight exposure than a child living in Manchester in the UK.

In terms of the measurements used to determine the level of vitamin D in the blood; most doctors will say that 30ng/ml (nanogram per milliter) is fine; however, consistent with other authorities on the subject, Cannell believes that it should be 50ng/ml or more. So ask to see the measurements.

Whilst taking the higher dose of 5,000iu for adults and adolescents is considered safe; because we metabolize it differently, in rare instances an overdose has caused problems. This is why it is important to get tested on a periodic basis. If in doubt, consult a reputable qualified nutritional practitioner or doctor for guidance.

Important note

Before purchasing a suitable supplement, I would strongly suggest that you seek advice from a reputable manufacturer or your doctor, since not all authorities agree on the dosage level for children and adults. You would also need to take into account variables such as your geographical location, how much time is spent outdoors and diet. A list of manufacturers are listed at the end of this book under 'Useful Information'. Moreover, not all experts on the subject will agree with the aforementioned dosages for children and adults.

Summary

A properly planned vegetarian diet can help to maintain and promote health, providing it is balanced as illustrated in the aforementioned Child B's diet, which is fairly close to an internationally recognized blueprint for health. Bear in mind, however, that supplementation with vitamin B12 and vitamin D3, may be essential. The benefits for your child may include:

- Probable reduced incidence of certain cancerous conditions, such as bowel and stomach cancer

- Better weight regulation

- Increased and sustained energy levels as a result of a steady level of blood-sugar

- Reduced incidence of heart and circulatory problems later in life

- Reduced incidence of mood swings and greater ability to concentrate due to steady blood sugar levels

- Improved immune function

- Greater resistance to illness

12

The Real Food Experience

Recently, I watched a TV show about school dinners and the importance of educating children about the origins of their food as well as making healthy choices. At one point the children were asked to identify certain fruits and vegetables. It was shocking to see that many could not even recognize the most basic produce; even vegetables like cabbages and carrots.

The fact is, these children are so used to living on food that comes out of packets that they are oblivious to what the original vegetable actually looks like, let alone what it is called or where it was grown.

Of course, many would argue that there must be a place within the school curriculum which addresses this issue; and some schools, to their credit, are setting about the task with great enthusiasm.

When I walk into such a school I get the feeling that all the teachers, and a lot of the parents for that matter, have embraced the whole concept of educating the pupils about healthy eating. This is reflected in a cross-curricular approach, which includes everything from organic gardening, science, food technology, PE, and personal, social, health education (PSHE).

School dinner ladies have been brought into the process, both as educators and providers of healthier food options. For the lucky schools that have an area of land where fruits and vegetables can be grown, it is wonderful to see the pupils getting involved in the growing and harvesting process. It is even better when their carefully tended produce ends up on a dinner plate in the school canteen. Even schools that have no growing area can always grow some produce in pots and other containers, so that this aspect of the curriculum can always feature to a lesser or greater degree. Look at a typical daily menu at one of these schools and you get the impression that they are 'putting their money where their mouth is', if you'll excuse the pun. Ok, to be honest, some of the menus I have looked at still leave a lot to be desired; but I for one am not too worried, because I figure that some improvements are better than none. Anyway, once healthier options have been included, more can be introduced as the whole healthier eating concept gathers momentum.

Parent Power

Let's face it, whatever influence schools may have on the health education of our children, we, as parents, can have the greatest influence on their development; especially if we are prepared to show them a good example in terms of healthy eating. However, this doesn't have to begin and end at the dinner table. It's really all about developing an awareness and respect for nature and our place within the grand order of things.

Modern feeding habits do not exactly encourage such awareness. In fact, conversely, the so-called Western style of eating, with its reliance upon packaged and sanitized foods, detaches our children from nature; and when you are detached from nature, you are detached from the very source of good health. Therefore, I always maintain that parents have a big responsibility towards their children to nurture a healthy respect for 'Mother earth'. In this way, children learn to appreciate their place within the whole ecosphere.

There are lots of ways that we can encourage such a healthy awareness in our children, and hopefully you will find some of the following ideas useful:

- Arrange a visit to a 'pick your own' farm in your area. There is no better way of learning about how fruits and vegetables are grown.

- Try to visit an organic farm. Taking your child to such an environment helps to foster an understanding of how crops can be grown without harming local wildlife, and it is easier for him/her to appreciate the importance of living in harmony with nature.

- Attempt to get your child involved in preparing and cooking food. Even very young children can become safely involved to some degree, e.g. helping to mix pastry in a hand-mixing bowl.

- Grow your own fruits and vegetables – if you have the time, inclination and even a small patch of garden; then try to get your child involved in growing some of your own produce. Children of all ages can get involved in the growing and harvesting process; even if it is only doing some occasional watering. They will also benefit from being able to eat the delicious home-grown produce too!

- Introduce your child to appropriate literature on the subject of healthy eating. There are some good books on the market, so look around.

13

Super Plants!

This chapter is all about plants that have a special reputation for healing and for boosting health. They are equally good for adults and children, and an increasing number of parents are becoming interested in how they can be used to boost their child's health and to help increase their resistance to illness.

Echinacea

Echinacea is wild flower with daisy-like purple colored blossoms, also known as the purple-cone flower. Native to the USA, it was used for centuries by the Plains tribes to heal wounds and counteract the venom from snakebites. It has also been used for many years as an all-round infection fighter and immune booster.

Echinacea is used to increase resistance to colds, influenza and infections in general. It works by stimulating various cells in the body's immune system that act as key weapons in the fight against invading organisms. It has been shown to kill bacteria, viruses, fungi and other harmful microbes.

How to take it

Echinacea comes in a variety of forms, including capsules, tablets and as a tincture. I think that the tincture is easier to use with children since you can add the drops to fruit juice, which helps to disguise the flavor. I would recommend that you choose a good quality brand such as A. Vogel/Bioforce.

Dosage

For children between 6 and 12 years old, it recommended that

7 drops are taken 2-3 times daily in a small amount of water or apple juice. Children over 12 years old should take 15 drops 2-3 times daily.

Possible side effects

No known side effects have been reported at recommended doses; however if your child is allergic to flowers in the daisy family it is best to avoid the use of this herb.

Spirulina

This is a form of freshwater algae which grows on the surface of freshwater lakes in places such as India and Hawaii. The algae is harvested and dried into powder. It can then be packaged and sold in its powdered from; or alternatively, made into tablets.

Spirulina is an easily digested whole food which is a great source of antioxidants such as beta carotene, in addition to all the essential amino acids. In fact, with regard to protein, it consists of a whopping 60% protein. It is also an amazing 58 times richer in iron than spinach.

Dosage

Children should take 2 x 500mg tablets or 2g of the powder per day. Add the powder to smoothies or mix with apple juice in a shaker.

Possible side effects

Providing the recommended dosage is observed, no side effects have been observed.

Garlic

Garlic belongs to the onion family which includes chives, onions, leeks and shallots. Whilst possessing the therapeutic value of onions, it is much more powerful. Garlic has been renowned as a health food for hundreds of years.

Garlic was valued in mediaeval times as a natural protector against infectious diseases. It was used to both ward off and clear bacterial infections. During the First World War garlic was revered by the Russian army for its infection-fighting qualities; so much so, that it was referred to as the Russian penicillin.

Most of the plant's therapeutic properties are derived from its sulfur compounds, of which there are more than 100. When the bulb is chewed or crushed, one of these sulfur compounds, alliin is converted to allicin, the chemical that is responsible for garlic's strong odor and health properties.

Garlic is also known to significantly lower blood cholesterol and can help to prevent atherosclerosis (hardening of the arteries). It also helps to prevent blood clots and has been shown to possess anti-cancer properties, particularly in the prevention of colon cancer.

Dosage
Garlic is most effective in its raw state, but to be honest, most children wouldn't appreciate having it chopped up and added to their salads. However, all is not lost since it can also be added to cooked dishes such as soups or casseroles, in addition to home-made salad dressings, such as French dressing. Failing this, providing your child is old enough to swallow them, I would suggest that you try giving him/her garlic tablets or capsules. However, try to choose supplements that contain around 400mcg of allicin per tablet or capsule.

Possible side effects
If high doses are taken, then it can cause diarrhea, intestinal gas and indigestion. The odor is also detectable on the breath and body through the pores.

Peppermint
Peppermint is a potent aromatic herb which herbalists have used

for centuries in order to relieve indigestion, colds and headaches. I particularly recommend it for its ability to soothe the digestive system.

It works by relaxing the intestinal muscles helping to dispel cramping and gas. This antispasmodic effect also means that it is great for alleviating irritable bowel syndrome; a complaint that is characterized by abdominal pain, and alternating bouts of constipation and diarrhea. Moreover, the menthol in peppermint stimulates the production of gastric juices and bile from the liver, thus aiding digestion. It is, of course, well known for its ability to freshen the breath.

Dosage

For nausea and irritable bowel syndrome it is best to give your child enteric-coated capsules (unless they are too young to swallow capsules of course). The capsules ensure that the oil of peppermint is released where it does the most good, which is in the large and small intestine.

To relieve trapped gas and indigestion you can give your child peppermint tea, to which a little honey can be added if desired. You can also purchase peppermint oil in bottled form from many health food shops. I prefer the Japanese oil of peppermint, which is very good. Add a few drops of the oil to hot or cold water and sip slowly. Children usually find it very soothing.

Possible side effects

In the recommended doses, peppermint has no side effects. Some very rare instances of skin rashes and indigestion caused by enteric-coated oil capsules have been reported.

Aloe Vera

Aloe vera looks a bit like a cactus, but it actually belongs to the lily family of plants. The leaves contain a cool soothing gel which has been used to treat burns and minor wounds for many years. The juice which is extracted from the plant is also used to sooth and heal the digestive system. In fact, whether used externally or internally, aloe vera is highly revered by herbalists and other therapists for its excellent healing properties.

Probably the reason why it is so effective in healing is because it contains a compound called bradykinase, which reduces pain and swelling. Some studies have indicated that aloe vera has anti-bacterial, anti-viral and anti-fungal properties. It also helps to boost the immune system. Aloe Vera gel is a wonderful method of alleviating and soothing sunburn when applied to your child's skin.

Dosage
For burns you can apply the gel repeatedly, as required to bring about relief.

For internal use you should follow the instructions on the bottle for child dosage. I would, however, recommend one capful twice per day in a little fruit juice.

Possible side effects
Poor quality juice may contain fragments of a substance known as aloe latex, which is the result of poor processing of the aloe vera plant. Therefore, if your child experiences diarrhea or loose stools after drinking the juice, then dispense with the particular brand that you are using and switch to one that is guaranteed to be processed to a high standard.

Apple Cider Vinegar
Cider vinegar is made by the fermentation of apples and the fermented fruit acid that is produced contains a host of vitamins and minerals, including potassium, magnesium, calcium, iron, trace minerals and a substance called pectin. The interesting thing about pectin is that it is a type of fiber which is known to

attach itself to cholesterol globules and remove any excess from the body. Cider vinegar also contains malic acid, which, not surprisingly, is found in apples. This type of acid is recognized by the body as a natural compound and it is much better than other harsh types of acid such as acetic, which can be irritating to the lining of the digestive system. Cider vinegar has a reputation as a powerful cleansing food as it breaks down mucous and phlegm in the body. It is also thought to be good for joints, and I would recommend it for children and adults who participate in regular sporting activities.

Dosage
I would recommend 2 to 3 tablespoonfuls per day, added to soups or casseroles. It is also excellent when pickling vegetables such as beetroot.

Possible side effects
Providing that your child exhibits no obvious adverse reaction to cider vinegar, then it is safe to use within the recommended dosage.

14

Juicy Kids!

Generally speaking, kids tend to like juices, especially the sweet tasting fruit juices. Indeed, these can be very health-promoting for your child; however, it is important not to forget the nutritional value of drinking vegetable juices, or fruit and vegetable combinations.

In fact, if your child gets into the habit of consuming freshly-made fresh juices on a regular basis, this will benefit his/her immune system, and provide an abundance of vitamins, minerals, phytochemicals and enzymes, all of which are rapidly absorbed by the body.

Freshly-made juices are not to be confused with the shop bought juices from supermarkets and health food shops. Those kinds of juices do have some nutritional value; however, their enzyme content will be greatly diminished since enzymes deteriorate rapidly from the moment the fruit or vegetable has been juiced.

The shop bought variety of juice will also be lacking in vitamins and minerals compared to the freshly-made type, since, again, vitamins and minerals diminish with time. What's more, if the juice has been pasteurized to extend its shelf-life, the heat from the pasteurization process will have destroyed all of the enzymes and a significant amount of the other nutrients. In stark contrast, freshly-made juices lose little of the nutrient value, providing they are consumed within 10 to 15 minutes after extraction. Such juices can provide a wonderful daily, easily absorbed health cocktail for your child that takes only about 25 minutes for the nutrients from a freshly-made juice to absorb into the bloodstream.

What is Juicing?

Now, this might seem like a silly question, but the fact is, lots of people get mixed up between juicing and blending. The simple explanation is as follows: when we juice an apple or carrot, the juicer opens up the cell walls of the plant, allowing the juice to escape. In other words, the juice is separated from the fiber. This juice is then channeled out of the machine where it can be collected in a jug or other receptacle. At the same time, the pulp or fibrous waste is channeled out in to a different container. The juice is then drunk either immediately or can be stored in the fridge for consumption later.

As I've already stated, it's best to consume a freshly-made juice within 10 to 15 minutes after it is extracted. The pulp is either discarded, or some people use it to make purees, soups, or stock.

By comparison, when we blend a fruit or vegetable, we are simply placing it in a blender (sometimes referred to as a liquidizer or smoothie maker) and breaking it down to a liquid. The difference is that the fiber is still present and you drink this along with the juice.

This is essentially what happens when we make a smoothie. Now, I'm not saying that smoothies aren't good; just that when we consume 100% juice without the fiber, its goodness is absorbed with hardly any effort on the part of the digestive system. In fact, in this way, we can absorb much larger amounts of health-giving nutrients into the blood stream very quickly indeed. This is why most of these detoxification retreats people go to base their detoxification programmes on the daily consumption of generous amounts of juices; including so-called green juices, which include green leafy vegetables, said to be the most health-promoting.

Of course, I am often confronted with the question: what about the lost fiber when we juice fruits and vegetables? Fiber is definitely a healthy part of a balanced diet and essential for the digestive system; however, providing our children are eating a fiber-rich healthy diet, the fiber discarded in the juicing process is not really an issue.

Choosing Your Juicer

The juicer that most people purchase is the centrifugal type. This consists of a powerful motor which drives a plate with blades. This plate is driven at a high speed and its cutting action separates the juice from the fiber. The juice is then flung against a bowl-shaped sieve and then channeled out of the machine. At the same time, the fiber is ejected through another channel. These juicers are very efficient and are capable of juicing quite large volumes of fruits and vegetables very quickly. The latest models have a wide feeding spout which allows you to juice whole apples and other large items. You can even include green leafy vegetables such as kale or spinach.

The only disadvantage associated with using this type of juicer is that because of the high speed extraction process, some heat is generated which will destroy some of the nutrients, including enzymes. This also happens due to the juice being mixed with the oxygen in the air, which has a similar destructive action. However, the juice is still of a high nutritional value.

TOP TIP!

When selecting a juicer opt for one that is easy to take apart for cleaning purposes. Also, if choosing a centrifugal type of juicer, choose one that has at least a 750w motor.

The other main type of juicer is the masticating juicer. You may have seen this type in these juice bars where they are used to make wheatgrass juice. They contain an auger which slowly crushes the fruit, vegetable or leafy greens, forcing the resulting juice through a cone-shaped sieve. The pulp is ejected at the end of the machine and comes out looking like a sausage. Although you have to chop the fruits or vegetables into smaller pieces to feed into the machine, and despite the fact it is slower; I do prefer this type of juicer because the quality of the juice is better; largely due to the fact that it involves less exposure to heat and air in the juicing process. Consequently, the nutrient level in the juice is greater when we use this type of juicer. Also, because the produce is crushed, more juice is extracted from the fiber resulting in more juice and less wastage. Some of the latest masticating juicers are even more efficient and can juice fruits and vegetables more quickly.

Masticating juicers are also capable of juicing wheatgrass. Wheatgrass are the young shots that grow from wheat seeds. It can be grown in soil-filled trays and as the name suggests, resembles grass in appearance. When it reaches around 6-8 inches high you can feed it into the machine and it produces the juice, which is exceptionally high in nutrients and chlorophyll. This type of juice is said to be highly detoxifying and nutritious, and for this reason it's best consumed in very small amounts. This usually means beginning with a couple of ounces a day, then building up to a few ounces daily.

Trays of ready grown wheatgrass can be purchased, or you can easily grow your own. To grow your own you simply soak about 200g of the wheat seeds in water for around six hours. Then drain off the water and evenly distribute the seeds over soil-filled seed trays. Water the seeds with just enough water to keep them moist and they will begin sprouting after a few days. Providing the sprouts are exposed to sunlight, they will turn green and soon grow to the requisite height. You don't need to keep them in strong sunshine; just enough daylight to develop normally. I would recommend that you purchase organically-grown seeds from a reputable supplier and also use organic soil for the trays. I have been doing this for the past year and the only tricky bit is making sure you keep a rotation going so that you have a steady supply of wheatgrass.

What About Cost?

You should be able to purchase a good centrifugal juicer for around £100 or $150 at the time of going to press. A masticating juicer is somewhat more expensive, and you may pay around £150 or $240 upwards.

Juicy Recipes for Kids

When it comes to juices, most people tend to think of commonly available juices such as carrot, apple, tomato, mixed vegetable, orange, grape and some of the more exotic ones such as mango and kiwi. Whereas these are very good, it's a good idea to be more versatile and use a wider range of ingredients. Here are some examples:

Omega Special

This juice provides children with essential healthy fats in the form of Omega 3 and Omega 6, which are excellent for healthy brain development.

2 whole apples
2 carrots
1 stick of celery (optional)
1 tsp of cold pressed flaxseed oil – a great source of essential
    fats

Method:
Juice the apples, carrots and celery. Stir-in the oil and mix well before drinking immediately. Serves 1.

As an alternative to the oil you can add a ½ scoop of the chia seed product MILA. See chapter 5, 'A Fat Lot of Good'.

Cool Kids

This is a great juice for hot sunny days as it contains cucumber which is very cooling. Cucumber is also a good supplier of important vitamins and minerals such as vitamin C and potassium.

½ cucumber
3 apples
2 sticks of celery
2 carrots

Method:
Juice all of the ingredients and garnish with a sprig of mint if desired. Serves 1-2.

Lemon Ginger Boost

Ginger is brilliant if you want to add a bit of zing to a juice. It's also great for the digestion and the circulation on cold winter days. It works well in a variety of juices; like this fruity combination.

½ inch piece ginger
¼ pineapple, peeled and sliced
1 apple or pear
½ lemon or 1 small lime

Method:
It's best to squeeze the lemon or lime in a citrus juice press in order to extract the juice. Then juice all of the other ingredients, adding the ginger last. Stir the resulting juice and serve. Serves 1.

NB. A sparkling version of this drink can easily be made by adding ½ glass of sparkling spring water to the juice. Kids love it!

Carrot and Soy Milk Surprise

You can add soy or almond milk to freshly juiced carrots for a refreshing creamy drink which kids love. This provides a high protein drink with an abundance of beta carotene which is what gives carrots their deep orange color. Beta carotene is converted by the body into vitamin A, which is great for maintaining a healthy immune system

.

3 medium size carrots
soy or almond milk to taste

Method:
Juice the carrots, stir-in the soy or almond milk and serve. Serves 1.

Green Power

This is one of my favorite juices because it is very good at detoxifying the body, protecting against pollution and providing an abundance of essential nutrients. This juice is so health-promoting because it includes a green, leafy vegetable which is rich in chlorophyll and other nutrients, such as magnesium and potassium.

Admittedly, your child may be put off by the green color; however, it tastes much better than it looks due to the apple juice it contains. If preferred, you can substitute the apple with carrot, which will also provide the sweetness required to make this juice palatable.

1 – 2 apples
2 sticks of celery
1/3 cucumber
a handful of spinach, kale or green cabbage

Method:

If you are using a centrifugal juicer, with the machine switched off, place the apples into the feeding spout first; then add the green, leafy vegetable, followed by the cucumber. Switch on the machine and use the plunger to force the vegetables through.

Jason Vale, otherwise known as the 'Juicemaster', calls this a sandwich, with the filling being the green leaves in the middle. By juicing the vegetables in this way, the maximum juice can be extracted from the green leaves. Finally, you juice the celery and stir the collected juice before drinking. If you use vegetables that have been stored in the fridge, the resulting cool tasting juice becomes more palatable to children. Failing this, add some crushed ice-cubes from the freezer.

NB. If you are using a masticating juicer you can simply juice all of the ingredients in any order, since this type of juicer is designed to deal with green leaves as well as all kinds of fruits and vegetables. Serves 1.

Blood Builder!

Beetroot is rich in iron which makes it a great blood builder. It is also one of the most powerful detoxifying vegetables for the liver, which is why you should only use the juice in small amounts, before gradually increasing the quantity used.

1 medium beetroot
2 apples
1 carrot
1 stick of celery

Method:

Simply scrub or peel the beetroot and carrot, then juice all of the ingredients and serve. Serves 1.

Fruity Spice

2 apples
1 tsp of mixed sweet spices
1 lime

Method:
Peel the lime, leaving on the pith. Juice together with the apples and sprinkle with the sweet spices. Serves 1.

Give Me Five!
This juice is packed full of vitamins and minerals and is very good for the digestion.

2 carrots
2 sticks of celery
1 small beetroot
2 tomatoes
1/3 medium size fennel

Method:
Juice all of the vegetables and serve with ice-cubes for a very refreshing drink. Serves 1-2.

Popeye

2 apples
2 carrots
handful of baby spinach
¼ of a cucumber

Method:
Use the method as described above for the green power juice, feeding the apples first into the juicer. Serves 1.

Vegetable Cocktail

This juice is similar to the mixed vegetable juices that you can purchase in cartons and bottles. However, this home-made version is much healthier for you and your children due to its content of enzymes and other nutrients.

1/2 cucumber
2 carrots
3 sticks of celery
3 tomatoes
1 beetroot
½ yellow pepper – deseeded and sliced
pinch of cayenne pepper (optional)

Method:
Simply juice all of the ingredients and add the sea salt and cayenne pepper if desired. Stir well and serve. Serves 1-2.

Banana Blend

1 peach
1 cup of strawberries or raspberries
1 pear
½ medium mango
1 banana

Method:
Deseed the peach and mango and juice along with the straw-berries / raspberries and pear. Pour the juice into a blender and blend with the banana and a handful of ice-cubes. This juice is a big favorite with kids. Serves 1-2.

Citrus Surprise

This juice is very refreshing, especially when served at breakfast time. It is a good source of vitamin C, which is good for your child's immune system.

2 oranges
2 apples

Method:
Peel the oranges leaving on the pith. Juice with the apples and serve. Serves 1.

Beta Booster!

Not only is carrot juice a great tasting juice in its own right, it is a wonderful source of beta carotene. Beta carotene is very good for your child's immune system as well as helping to promote the health of the skin and eyes.

5 medium size carrots

Method:
Juice the carrots and drink within 15 minutes if possible in order to benefit from its nutrients. This home-made version is far superior in flavor compared to the bottled varieties on sale in shops. Serves 1.

Probiotic Power!

A Probiotic is just another name for the healthy bacteria that live in the gut. These health bacteria help to keep the gut healthy, aid in digestion, support the immune system and even make certain nutrients such as some B vitamins. You can purchase acidophilus powder in health food shops or pharmacies that can be added to freshly extracted juices, such as the one below:

1 apple
1 pear
1 carrot
½ tsp of acidophilus powder

Method:
Juice the fruit and carrot and stir in the acidophilus powder before serving. Serves 1.

Tropical Taster
Your child will love this delightful mix of tropical fruits.

1/3 pineapple
2 kiwi fruit
½ mango
handful of grapes
1 cup of ice-cubes

Method:
Deseed the mango and juice with the other fruits. Blend the ice-cubes in a blender and add to the juice. Serve with a sprig of mint (optional). Serves 1-2.

Liver Booster
This is a good juice for supporting the liver as well as reducing heavy metals.

1 lemon, peeled
1 apple
1 carrot
2 cabbage leaves
1 beetroot
½ inch of ginger
1 tsp of chlorella powder

Method:
Juice the fruits and vegetables. Pour off the juice and stir-in the chlorella powder and mix thoroughly. Serves 1.

Skin Cleanser
This juice is great for children who suffer from acne and other skin problems.

1 apple
2 carrots
2 sticks of celery
½ beetroot
2 cabbage leaves
½ inch of ginger

Method:
Juice all of the ingredients and drink immediately. Serves 1.

The Refresher
This juice is good for stomach upsets and is very refreshing.

1/3 cucumber
2 sticks of celery
2 red apples
3 inch slice of fresh pineapple
½ cup of fresh mint leaves

Method:
If using a centrifugal type of juicer; with the juicer switched off, place an apple in the feeding spout; then add the mint leaves, followed by the other apple. Switch on the juicer and juice these ingredients followed by the cucumber and the celery. If using a masticating juicer you can juice the ingredients in any order as it can easily deal with the mint leaves separately. Serves 1.

Orange Energizer

This juice is a great energizer and a good source of nutrients.

2 oranges, peeled
2 broccoli florets
½ cantaloupe melon
1 carrot
a handful of spinach
½ cup of sunflower or alfalfa sprouts

Method:
If using a centrifugal juicer juice use the sandwich method with the spinach leaves and alfalfa providing the filling. If using a masticating juicer, juice ingredients in any order. Serves 1-2.

Acid-Buster

This is a wonderful juice for neutralizing excess acids in the body; particularly after excessive eating, for example after a party celebration for your child's birthday.

2 sticks of celery
1 apple
1 lemon, peeled
1/3 cucumber
1 red radish
3 inch slice of pineapple
½ inch of ginger

Method:
Juice all of the ingredients and serve with crushed ice (optional). Serves 1.

Germ Buster!
This juice is antiseptic and acts as a natural antibiotic.

2 apples
1 carrot
a handful of spinach
½ inch ginger
¼ red onion

Method:
Not all children will find this a palatable juice. You may wish to dilute it with water.

Smoothies

When it comes to healthy eating, smoothies have their place in terms of contributing towards your child's daily intake of fruits. There are many different smoothie recipes and here are a few that you might like to try:

Banana, Pineapple and Kiwi
This is a delightful mix of tropical flavors coupled with the creaminess of the yoghurt.

125g of bio-yoghurt or soy yoghurt
1 banana
¼ pineapple
1 kiwi fruit (peeled)

Method:
Remove the skin from the pineapple and kiwi fruit. Cut the pineapple into chunks. Place all of the ingredients into the blender and blend until creamy and smooth. Serves 1.

Omega Special

By adding a small amount of a cold-pressed balanced oil formula containing Omega 3 and Omega 6 healthy fats, you will be combining the nutritious elements of the fruits along with the essential fats so beneficial to young children.

1 pear
1 apple
1 banana
1 cup of soy or almond milk
1 tbsp of Omega blend oil or ½ scoop of MILA (see chapter 5)

Method:
Blend all of the fruits along with the soy or almond milk. If using MILA, add this and blend for a few seconds. If using the oil, drizzle it into the mixture and stir thoroughly. Drink immediately so that the essential fats in the oil do not become damaged by exposure to the light and air. Serves 1.

Berry in a Hurry

For a quickly prepared antioxidant-rich smoothie, try this nutritious berry packed drink:

125g bio yoghurt
1 cup of blueberries
2 plums
1 cup of strawberries

Method:
Remove the stones from the plums. Blend all of the ingredients and serve. Serves 1.

Coconut Dream

Kids love this smoothie with its fruity flavors combined with the fresh taste of coconut.

3 apricots
1 peach
1 kiwi fruit
1 medium-sized mango
½ can of coconut milk

Method:
Peel the mango and peach, then remove their stones and cut into pieces; peel the kiwi fruit and cut into slices. Blend with the apricots adding the coconut milk until creamy and smooth. Serves 1.

Banana, Peach and Strawberries

Children love the combined flavors of this creamy smoothie:

1 banana
10 strawberries
1 peach
3 tbsp of bio-yoghurt or soy milk

Method:
Remove the stone from the peach and cut into chunks. Cut the banana into slices. Put all of the fruit into the blender and add the yoghurt or soy milk last of all. Serves 1.

Carrot Smoothie

By utilizing your juicer and blender you can produce this smoothie which is a great source of beta carotene and vitamin C.

1 apple
1 banana
2 medium size carrots
1 pear
1 kiwi fruit
125g of bio yoghurt or soy yoghurt

Method:
Juice the carrots in your juicer. Blend the fruits and yoghurt together in the blender. Add the carrot juice and mix well before serving. Serves 1.

Green Smoothie
1 cup frozen berries
2 handfuls of spinach
400 mls of rice milk or almond milk

Method:
Blend all of the ingredients together and serve.

15

Pollution Protection for Kids

Environmentalists tell us that if we continue to pollute our planet at the present rate, then irreversible damage will be a reality within 30 or 40 years.

Most of us tend to think of pollution as a modern problem. However, it's been going on as a direct result of mankind's activities for hundreds of years. For instance, during medieval times, the river Thames which flows through the city of London was so polluted by all of the sewage being dumped into it that it became a real health hazard. Nor was pollution confined to the rivers of big cities such as New York, Chicago and London.

Air pollution also posed a big threat to people residing in large suburban conurbations. Again, London, England, was one of the worst places for smog. Smog, as the name suggests, is a combination of smoke (largely from chimneys) and fog.

Until the 12th century, most Londoners burned wood for fuel. However, as the forests shrank and wood became scarce, Londoners began using sea-coal in order to fuel their fires and their factories. Sea-coal was plentiful, but it didn't burn that efficiently, resulting in large volumes of smoke being produced. This acrid smoke mixed with the natural fog that hung over London, forming dangerous smog. This situation persisted until 1952, when a four-day fog killed roughly 4,000 Londoners. It was after this that British Parliament enacted the Clean Air Act in 1956, thereby reducing the burning of coal.

The modern equivalent of this would be cities such as Los Angeles, where fog combines with car exhaust fumes to form 'smog'. People exposed to this kind of air pollution can develop lung problems such as asthma and bronchitis.

As a result of so-called global warming, we are being forced to seriously consider ways of reducing carbon emissions from vehicle exhausts, factories and our overall use of energy. Car manufacturers now have to design new so-called hybrid cars that run on more than one source of energy; or in the case of electric cars, on electricity driven motors. Undoubtedly, there are some positive changes afoot; however, both adults and children are constantly being exposed to a vast array of chemicals on an everyday basis.

A lot of these chemicals come from modern farming, for example pesticides, nitrates, herbicides and fungicides. Others get into the environment as a result of industrial processes. For instance, mercury, a highly toxic metal that can adversely affect the nervous system, is sometimes present in the livers of fish, such as tuna. Dioxins, which are chemicals found in some plastic water bottles and PCB's, otherwise known as polychlorinated hydrocarbons, also present a hazard to humans as they can get into the food chain. In addition, a number of radioactive materials are sometimes detectible in the environment; for example from atomic bomb testing and due to the use of the depleted uranium weaponry that was used in Iraq.

Although the body has a number of coping mechanisms which come into play when these foreign substances enter the body, we have now reached a situation in which the body's main organ of detoxification, namely, the liver, is encountering chemicals that are new to it. Fortunately, the liver is a very complex organ that has at its disposal hundreds of enzymes which act upon pollutants in order to render them harmless to the body. However, if the capacity of the body to detoxify is overworked, it is thought that many toxins are stored in tissues, such as fat cells in order to isolate them. This is the body's attempt to protect other vital cells from their harmful effects.

All of this sounds pretty grim, especially when we must acknowledge that it is impossible to insulate our precious children in such a polluted world. Nevertheless, do not despair, because apart from taking steps to minimize exposure to pollutants, there is much that can be done nutritionally and through exercise that will help to protect ourselves and our offspring.

How Organically-Grown Unprocessed Foods Help to Protect Children from the Effects of Chemicals!

Now, I stress here the importance of organically-grown produce, since the consumption of such foods automatically reduces the intake of chemicals into the body. The less chemicals that your child's body has to cope with through food, the more efficiently he or she will be able to deal with environmental chemicals; for example from air pollution.

The nutrients present in natural foods are required to make the enzymes needed by the liver to detoxify toxins, and if your child has a high nutrient intake as a result of eating healthy foods, then his/her liver will cope with pollution better than your average junk food eating kid! When a child is fed on junk foods, not only does the liver not receive the raw materials that it needs to deal with harmful chemicals from pollution, it also has to deal with the chemical additives found in the foods themselves! And besides that, the body often has to use some of its own supplies of nutrients in order to digest the likes of white sugar, white flour and all products made from them. Basically, it's a no win situation.

Heavy Metal Protection Plan

Following the general healthy eating advice in this book will help to protect both adults and children from the effects of heavy metals. It would also be advisable to implement the following measures:

- Make use of minerals that counteract the toxicity of heavy metals like magnesium, selenium and zinc; these are available in children's vitamin/mineral formulas – see below.

- These nutrients are also available from green leafy vegetables, fruits and seeds.

- Include in your child's diet foods rich in pectin which bind the toxic metals allowing them to be excreted from the body. Pectin is found in fresh fruits such as apples, bananas, pears and plums.

- Include foods such as pulses, seeds, white meat, fish and whole grains.

- Give your child a broad spectrum vitamin and mineral supplement appropriate for their age – see recommended supplements at the end of this book.

- Consider using the naturally-occurring mineral zeolite to help remove heavy metals from the body. See the radiation protection plan shown later in this chapter.

HEAVY METALS AND BEHAVIORAL PROBLEMS

The Center for disease control and Prevention in the United States has stated that lead poisoning remains the most common environmental health issue affecting children in the USA.

A 2007 study in Michigan State indicated that blood levels of heavy metals deemed to be in the safe range, were linked with the occurrence of Attention Deficit Disorder (ADD) and Attention Deficit Hyperactivity Disorder (ADHD).

Heavy metals can be removed from the body using chelating minerals or by using the volcanic mineral, zeolite.

The following information table highlights the different types of pollution and the action required to reduce your child's exposure:

TYPE OF POLLUTION	POSSIBLE EFFECTS	MINIMIZING EXPOSURE
Exhaust fumes	Asthma, lung irritation bronchitis	Where possible, avoid busy roads and highways; choose quieter routes whenever practicable. If you live near a busy road close your windows at night. If you are concerned about air quality in your home consider installing an air purifier.
Aerosol sprays	Asthma, lung irritation	Avoid using aerosol sprays such as deodorants, air fresheners and insecticide sprays in confined spaces where children may be exposed. Open windows to circulate air and help to dispel air-borne chemicals from the spray.
Tobacco smoke	Asthma, bronchitis, increased susceptibility to lung cancer	Thankfully, most public places in countries such as the USA, Australia and the UK are smoking-free zones these days. If you smoke, avoid smoking in confined places where children are present.

| Pesticides, herbicides, fungicides | Unknown, but may be implicated in various cancers, eye abnormalilites and infertility. | Opt for organically grown foods whenever possible. Wash conventionally grown produce thoroughly and peel the likes of apples, pears and root vegetables such as carrots. |

Heavy metals

| Mercury | Damaging to the nervous system | If your child is vaccinated check for vaccines containing mercury, as this has been associated with an increase in cases of autism, ADHD and nerve damage. A substance called thimerosal is used as a preservative in vaccines and this contains mercury. Reduce tuna consumption to twice per week. Opt for mercury-free dental fillings. |
| Lead | Damaging to the nervous system | Avoid exposure to solvents and lead-containing paints. If your drinking water is channeled through lead piping (less common these days) ensure that you run the cold water for a few minutes first thing in the morning. This helps to dissipate the lead particles that can accumulate during the night. |

Aluminum	Possible link with Alzheimer's disease; neurotoxin	Avoid use of aluminum cookware such as aluminum pans. Also, aluminum foil. Scrutinize labels on products such as anti-acid remedies, toothpaste and bakery products due to the additives used in their manufacture. Avoid unfiltered tap water.
Cadmium	Similar to lead as it can damage the nervous system affecting brain development. May be linked with behavioral problems.	Found in cigarette smoke, so avoid whenever possible.

Water

Fluoride	Controversy reigns over the use of fluoride in drinking water. Has been linked with fluorosis (mottling of teeth) when used in excess of 2 parts per million.	Whenever possible use filtered water for drinking and cooking purposes as most of the fluoride will be extracted in the filtering process. Most toothpastes and some mouthwashes contain fluoride, unless you opt for natural fluoride-free products.

Chlorine	Unproven to be harmless to health. Added to water supplies to eradicate harmful microorganisms. Can react with substances such as peat, forming the toxic substance chloroform, associated with some cancers.	Use filtered or spring water instead of tap water whenever possible.
Nitrates	Sometimes found in water supplies due to drainage from nitrate fed crops. Can form nitrosamines which are known to be carcinogenic.	Opt for filtered water or spring water known to be free from excessive nitrates.
Radiation	Exposure from a variety of sources can lead to greater susceptibility to cancers and immune system damage.	Avoid exposure to excessive use of x-rays whenever feasible. Adhere to the radiation protection plan at the end of this chapter.

Water – Making the Right Choice

In view of the fact that water often contains a number of pollutants, including heavy metals, nitrates, chlorine and fluoride, it is
a good idea to seek out cleaner sources. These may include the
following:

Bottled water

The majority of bottled waters come from water that has
filtered through several layers of rock. These rocks can act as
a filter which removes any contaminants, whilst at the same
time, minerals acquired from the rocks will influence the
water's mineral composition. For example, water that is
filtered through limestone is likely to be high in calcium.

Filtered water

Plumbed in water filters seem to be quite popular these days.
These are plumbed into the water supply of your house and
the filtered water is channeled through a separate tap.

The Filter itself contains carbon, which is great at filtering
out pollutants such as heavy metals and chlorine. They do
have to be changed regularly in order to avoid bacterial
growth and to ensure the efficiency of the filtration process.

If you don't want to go to the expense of paying for a
plumbed in water filter, I would suggest you buy a good
quality jug-type filter. The filters in these are also based on
carbon and do the same kind of job. Again, the filters must be
changed regularly.

Distilled water

Distilled water is probably the purest type of water; however,
it lacks any taste due to the fact that it is devoid of minerals as
a result of the distillation process. Despite this fact, I feel that
it is still preferable to drinking tap water.

Reverse osmosis filters

As far as removing impurities and bacteria are concerned, this type of filter is the most efficient. However, they are expensive and use up a lot of electricity.

Electromagnetic Fields

On those few occasions when we're unfortunate enough to suffer a power cut in our electricity supply, it becomes blatantly obvious just how dependant we are on this form of energy. In fact, a world devoid of washing machines, dishwashers, electric ovens, immersion heaters, televisions, computers or a cordless phone, would be unthinkable to most of us. Certainly, the advent of such technology has brought with it many benefits. Nevertheless, there is often a down side to such advancements, and this is no less true when we think of many everyday electrical devices found in our homes.

Whenever an electrical current flows an electromagnetic field is created. Such energy fields (EMFs for short) are being increasingly linked with disorders such as cancer and problems with the central nervous system; including dementia, Parkinson's disease and the chronic fatigue syndrome M.E.

Doctors and scientists world wide, have found evidence of a connection between EMFs and disease. However, there is some controversy surrounding such claims. Opposing views on this subject continue to dominate the media. A typical example might be a newspaper report which highlights a study on overhead power lines, which emit high levels of EMFs. The study indicates that there is a strong link between living near such power lines and the incidence of leukemia. The following week, it would not be unusual for that same newspaper to feature a study that claims the opposite to be true.

I suppose that what it comes down to is gathering as much information on the subject as possible and making an informed choice based upon that information. To be perfectly honest, in terms of the welfare of our children, I'd rather err on the side of caution whenever possible. If people had waited for conclusive proof that smoking cigarettes definitely causes lung cancer before giving up smoking, then the mortality rates would have been even more catastrophic.

When it comes to EMFs and other potential threats to health, such as genetically modified foods; I feel that it is not such a bad idea to be cautious. Besides, I have had too many parents say to me that the health of their son or daughter significantly improved after reducing their exposure to EMFs within their home. This might be something as simple as moving the position of their child's bed so that it was positioned further away from an electrical source; for example, an immersion heater, or a telephone base for a portable telephone.

Ok, so by this stage you could be forgiven for asking just how we are to eliminate all EMF's from our homes, offices, shops and literally everywhere. Well, it's true that we cannot entirely isolate ourselves or our children from modern technology; however, we can take some simple precautionary steps in order to minimize any negative effects from electrical appliances such as televisions and computers.

The following guide explains which specific appliances found in the home give off EMF's and other potentially harmful energy fields and how we can minimize their effects:

Bedside clock radio: These produce significant levels of magnetic fields.

Action Required: Locate mains-powered clocks a minimum of 1 meter from your child's bed-head. Battery powered clocks produce negligible fields, so they are a far safer option.

Bedside lights: These do give off EMFs and should be placed as far away as is practicable from the child's bed.

Action Required: Bedside lights should be switched off at the socket overnight to avoid unnecessary exposure to EMF's.

Computers: Most modern computers emit low levels of EMF's. Encourage your child to sit no closer than 50cm; and shut down and switch off the computer at the mains (not just leaving it on stand-by). This also saves energy.

Computer monitors (VDU): The old type of cathode ray tube type of VDUs, tend to emit high EMFs in addition to x-rays. However, these computer monitors are becoming obsolete. Long-term use of these types of screens is associated with headaches, anxiety, fatigue, irritability and eye strain. It is also known that cathode ray VDUs give off more EMFs at the back and the sides compared to modern flat screen computers.

Action Required: Always make sure that your child sits more than 1 meter away from the back of a VDU. Remember that magnetic fields can penetrate through walls, so take this into account when positioning VDUs in rooms adjacent to your child's bedroom or study area.

Laptop computers: When a mains adapter is used to power the laptop a high level of EMFs are produced.

Action Required: Whenever possible your child should use a laptop run on charged up battery power, not actually plugged in at the mains at time of use. . Using a laptop computer on a solid surface such as a desk, is preferable to your child using it on their lap due to the close proximity to the body.

Wi-Fi (wireless internet connections) these use radio waves just like cell phones. This communication across a wireless network is very much like a two-way radio. What happens is that a computer's wireless adapter translates data into a radio signal and transmits it using an antenna; then a wireless router receives the signal and decodes it. The router sends the signal to the internet using a wired ethernet connection.

Since the router uses mains electricity, it does produce EMFs. However, this aside, there is much debate as to the potential harmful affects of being exposed to the radio waves used in this type of technology; particularly where children are concerned.

In the UK, the director of the consumer group, **Powerwatch, Alasdair Philips**, has this to say about wi-fi in schools:

"Our brains and nervous systems work by using electrical signals. I believe these signals are being interfered with by exposure to this wi-fi radiation. Based on studies reporting effects experienced by people living near mobile phone masts, I would predict chronic fatigue, memory and concentration problems, irritability and behavior problems – exactly what we are seeing increasingly in our school pupils".

Action Required: Do not locate routers in bedrooms (a hall or landing would be better). Switch off routers when not in use and ensure your child avoids placing a laptop computer on their lap when using wi-fi.

Computer games: Games consoles usually use a mains transformer that plugs into a power socket. These emit a very high level of EMFs.

Action Required: It is important to unplug them when not in use. This is especially important if your child's bed is located near a transformer. It is better to keep computer games consoles away from the children's bedrooms, in a games room for example.

Cordless phones: Until quite recently cordless phones have not been mentioned in the same breath as mobile / cell phones in terms of potential risks. However, it is known that both the base unit and phone itself do emit microwave radiation. Although the radiation is lower than that produced by mobile/cell phones, we need to take into account that we tend to use cordless phones for longer periods; thus in the long-term the user may be subjecting the brain to greater amounts of microwave radiation.

Action Required: Use a telephone that plugs into a telephone socket in favor of a cordless phone. Failing this, try to limit the time your child uses a cordless phone and try to encourage them to use the speaker phone to avoid exposure close to their brain. Be aware that the base units for such phones can also emit microwave radiation; therefore, ensure that the base unit is positioned somewhere away from where your child sleeps or sits.

Mobile/cell phones: At the moment the jury is still out on mobile phones, although current research continues to provide evidence that microwave radiation may affect the brain, causing both short and long-term memory loss, headaches, confusion and even brain tumors.

Any health risk is likely to be increased where children's brains are concerned as they are still developing. A lot of evidence is anecdotal at present, but research on chicks and small mammals such as rats has revealed some disturbing evidence. The chicks were killed by radiation from mobile / cell phones, and mammals involved in these experiments showed definite signs of short-term memory loss.

Action Required: If your child uses a mobile phone try to stress the possible harmful effects and encourage them to use their phone sparingly and to send texts rather than calling whenever feasible. It would also be sensible for your child to use the speaker phone option whenever possible. Finally, it is preferable to carry the mobile phone in a bag rather than keeping it in a pocket.

Televisions: Color televisions give off quite high levels of EMFs from the sides and back of the TV.

Action Required: If possible, make sure that your child sits at least 2 meters away from the TV screen. Use of a remote control is to be encouraged since it means that your child doesn't need to be in close contact with the screen when changing channels. Put the television in a family lounge but not in the children's bedrooms. Since magnetic fields go through walls, give some thought to the positioning of the TV in relation to your child's bedroom and where they spend a lot of their time, such as a study or playroom. Switch the television set off at the mains, don't just leave it on stand-by as this uses more electricity and gives off constant EMF emissions.

Immersion heaters: The central heating pumps, heater and associated wiring, generate high EMFs.

Action Required: Ensure that your child's bed head is at least 1 meter from the location of an immersion heater, bearing in mind that EMFs can even travel through walls.

Microwave ovens: These produce high levels of EMFs and older ovens may leak microwave radiation.

Action Required: It's preferable to cook conventionally on a hob wherever possible. If you use a microwave in your cooking, avoid your child standing close to a working microwave oven. Preferably no closer than 2 meters away.

Hi-fi systems and i-Pod docking stations: Both of these can give off high levels of EMFs.

Action Required: Ensure that your child is not sleeping or sitting within 2 meters of these appliances.

Hairdryers: These create high magnetic fields and have been linked with the malfunction of the pineal gland found deep in the brain. This gland produces melatonin which appears to be connected with cancer protection and cell regeneration. It may be significant that melatonin increases during the night.

Action Required: If possible, children should avoid using a hairdryer after 6pm.

Washing machines/dishwashers: Both appliances give off high levels of EMFs.

Action Required: Whilst the appliances are operating, stay at least 1 meter away from them. Keep these appliances in a utility room if at all possible. In any case, ensure that children do not play in close proximity to such appliances.

Electricity pylons: EMFs are emitted from the overhead cables, not the towers themselves. The higher the voltage being transmitted through the cables, the greater the level of EMFs.

Some research has shown that the electric fields result in air ionization which in turn may include carcinogenic particles. The possible health risks associated with living in close proximity to electricity pylons is still the subject of much debate. Anecdotal evidence has linked health conditions such as headaches and disturbed sleep patterns with exposure to the electric fields; and research continues into increased rates of cancers, such as childhood leukemia, near pylons.

Action Required: It would appear that some people are more sensitive than others when it comes to exposure to EMFs. However, if you live in close proximity to overhead pylons and you suspect that your health or the health of your child is suffering in any way; the only option is to re-locate; although this may be not practicable for some people. If you fall into this category, it is important to implement the nutritional advice encompassed within this book.

Cellular phone base-stations and masts: Base stations and masts are known to emit a continuous stream of microwave radiation. Official agencies say that signals produced are not powerful enough to be dangerous. However, it would seem that our bodies do pick up the pulsing of these signals and evidence suggests that they can interfere with cellular processes; such as cell division.

Maximum fields from these masts at ground level are usually detectable between 30-100 meters away. The current practice of siting masts in school grounds is now giving great cause for concern and a number of campaigns in the USA and other technologically advanced countries are attempting to put a stop to this policy.

Some scientific reports have suggested that microwave radiation may cause leukemia, cataracts, brain tumors and heart conditions. In response to the mounting evidence, countries, such as New Zealand, are now adopting policies that state that cellular phone antennas should not be cited near schools in the future.

Radiation

We are all familiar with manmade radiation which has become an integral part of modern society. When you mention the word radiation most people think of nuclear power and X-Rays. However, in its broadest sense, 'radiation' refers to energy waves and light waves. Sunlight for example, is a source of radiation.

When ionizing radiation comes into contact with living tissue, it can cause damage. Non-ionizing radiation, such as radio waves, don't have this affect.

X-rays

The form of radiation that represents the greatest threat to health, known as ionizing radiation, comes from the likes of gamma rays and X-rays. Modern medicine still relies upon x-rays for medical and dental diagnostic purposes, and X-rays are also used routinely in airports in order to check luggage. Some exposure to X-rays is unavoidable; for example for detecting possible tooth decay or for possible bone fractures. Fortunately, new technology has resulted in lower doses for diagnostic purposes. Nevertheless, adopting the measures in the radiation protection plan in this chapter is a good idea.

Nuclear power stations

Like it or loathe it, nuclear power produces a significant amount of our electricity.

Of course, a lot of controversy still surrounds the safety of atomic power stations. This is hardly surprising in the light of what happened in the former USSR in 1986, when the nuclear power station at Chernobyl produced substantial nuclear fall-out when a reactor caught fire.

This caused air-borne fall-out which contaminated large areas of Europe, including Britain. This did cause some contamination of food supplies in these areas. Most of the contamination in the UK was confined to regions like Cumbria, Wales and Scotland

and affected mainly sheep. Subsequent restrictions were imposed on the sale of contaminated livestock, and to this day, as far as I am aware, the situation still has to be monitored.

The Chernobyl disaster resulted in an increasing lack of confidence in the nuclear power industry, especially in view of the adverse publicity associated with alleged radioactive leaks at power stations such as Sellafield in the UK and the partial core meltdown in a pressurized water reactor on Three Mile Island in Dauphin County, Pennsylvania. The latter resulted in the release of significant amounts of radioactive materials into the environment.

Personally, I could never be comfortable with the thought that radioactive waste from nuclear power stations is regularly discharged into our environment, including the seas around our shores. Unfortunately, as the Chernobyl disaster proved, radiation does not recognize boundaries. This was further highlighted in the late 1950s and early 1960s, when nuclear testing in the Pacific resulted in radioactive contamination around the world.

Tolerance levels
The consequences of exposure to high levels of radiation are well known as we will recall from the bombing of Hiroshima in Japan during the Second World War. Many people died of radiation sickness, and for many years after the nuclear explosions took place the occurrence of cancer and birth defects remained high. This is also evident in and around the Chernobyl area in the former Soviet Union; where, significantly, there is now a great demand for supplies of vitamin and mineral supplements which can help offset some of the effects of radioactive contamination.

Depleted uranium
Some authorities on the subject believe that unless another catastrophe occurs most of us will be exposed to much smaller

doses of radioactivity over a long period of time.

However, having said this, there is some concern about depleted uranium contamination around the world. Depleted uranium was used in munitions such as bombs, rockets and even bullets in both Gulf Wars. The inclusion of the depleted uranium provides a mighty punch, enabling the shells to penetrate tanks, concrete and so on.

As it penetrates it combusts and any human life on the receiving end is instantly incinerated.

From an environmental perspective, hundreds of tons of depleted uranium were used in Iraq during the course of both Gulf Wars. This has exposed thousands of troops and civilians to depleted uranium fall-out, and there is evidence that cancer rates and birth defects have markedly increased among the population of Iraq as well as in the troops serving in those wars.

Unfortunately, it appears that depleted uranium dust particles have contaminated other countries having been carried in the wind. Depending upon your geographical location, your exposure to this radioactive material will vary. However, it is a concern, especially in children, as they are more susceptible to the effects of radiation.

The good news is that we all have coping mechanisms within the body designed to protect us from low levels of radiation exposure. If this were not the case then as a species we would not have survived this long, since our primitive ancestors were exposed to low-level background radiation which is emitted from rocks, soil, food and water. Of course, such background radiation is still present in our modern day environment.

In addition to this we are also exposed to cosmic radiation from the sun and outer space. Much of this radiation is reduced by the time it reaches us, since the earth's atmosphere acts as a shield. However, the higher we are above sea level, the more radiation we are exposed to.

Bearing this in mind, it is estimated that the amount of

radiation that we are exposed to every time we fly, is the equivalent of one chest X-ray. For this reason, I feel that airplane pilots and stewardesses may be more at risk from radiation related illnesses. In this regard, research published in 2001, indicated that breast cancer among women flight attendants was found to be 30% higher than normal, and skin cancer among male attendants is twice as high as normal. These findings emerged from a study of 6,000 flight attendants in the United States. Other studies have concluded that male pilots have a higher incidence of colon, rectum, prostate and brain cancer than the rest of the population.

If your child accompanies you on frequent flights I would advise you to implement the radiation protection measures at the end of this section.

Radon
Radon gas is produced as a result of the radioactive decay of Uranium. It is a significant cause of human exposure to radiation, occurring mostly indoors. Uranium and radium, which is its decay product, is a natural component of soil and rocks and can be found in some wood, bricks and concrete. When these decay products are released into the atmosphere and subsequently inhaled, they settle in the lungs where they will emit radiation. Fortunately, in the open air, most of the radon gas is quickly dispersed. The problem arises when the gas builds up inside buildings since it can be released from the very soil and rocks upon which the building is built. Under such circumstances, the gas builds up and is inhaled over a period of time.

Surveys carried out in Britain have indicated that certain areas, such as the south-west of England, are more affected than others. Furthermore, areas with high levels of granite such as parts of Scotland and Wales are more likely to produce radon.

Getting tested

If you live in a high risk area you can contact your local Environmental Health Officer, who should be able to provide you with specific information about any potential risks associated with the location of your house. Sometimes tests are carried out where this is deemed to be justified.

If you reside in the USA, you can call the National Radon Information Line on:

1-800-SOS-RADON
1 (800) 767-7236
Australian residents should contact the
Australian Radiation and Nuclear Safety Agency
Email: info@arpansa.gov.au Tel: +61 3 9433 2211

The Radiation Protection Plan

When radioactive elements enter the body they are absorbed into the tissues. Some of these elements have an affinity for specific areas of the body.

Cesium 137, an end product of the atomic bomb tests in the Pacific, has an affinity for iodine. For this reason, cesium will build up in the thyroid gland, found in the throat, where plentiful iodine is needed to ensure normal thyroid function. What is amazing is that cesium levels in the thyroid can be reduced if an iodine-rich supplement such as kelp (a type of seaweed) is taken regularly. It is important to purchase kelp that is harvested from deep sea areas which should be relatively pollution-free. The uptake of iodine by the thyroid helps to exclude the radioactive cesium from being absorbed into the thyroid tissue.

The same story holds true with the radioactive element strontium 90, which has an affinity for calcium. Once inside the body it gravitates towards areas that are high in calcium, such as the skeleton.

We can protect ourselves from strontium if our diet is high in calcium. In the case of children, much of this calcium can come from a natural diet that is high in organic calcium, such as from green leafy vegetables, almonds and sesame seeds. In addition to this, parents would be wise to include a vitamin and mineral supplement recommended for children.

Important!
Always adhere to manufacturers recommendations on dosage with children's formulas. This is also important in relation to the number of powdered kelp or kelp tablets taken by children.

Protection from radiation
In order to protect ourselves and our children from the effects of radiation, we need to adopt the following strategy:

- Take steps to limit exposure to radiation wherever possible. For example, try to purchase food which is grown in mainly low-land areas; remembering that certain highland areas around the world were contaminated by radioactive fall-out.

- Give your child a good broad spectrum vitamin and mineral supplement recommended for children – see children's supplements at the end of this chapter.

- Ensure that your child adheres to a natural diet.

- Make good use of chlorophyll-rich foods such as broccoli, cabbage, sprouts, lettuce, spinach and kale. Chlorophyll is thought to exert a protective effect against radiation.

- Try sprouting your own nuts, seeds and grains. When sprouted they are rich in nutrients which may exert a protective affect. Many of these sprouts, such as sunflower, snow peas and broccoli, are also high in chlorophyll.

- Use kelp powder sparingly in soups and other cooked dishes. It is rich in iodine and other protective minerals.

- Give your child chlorella powder or tablets. Chlorella is believed to exert a protective affect against radiation and helps to eliminate it from the body. Avoid giving tablets to very young children in case of choking. Adhere to the manufacturers recommendations for dosage.

- If you have a juicer try to get your child into the habit of making at least one or two fresh organic fruit and vegetable juices each day. Drinking freshly prepared enzyme and nutrient rich juices daily can help protect you and your children from the effects of pollution; including low-level radiation.

- Consider using zeolite. As with heavy metal protection, this volcanic mineral has been shown to bind with radioactive materials such as depleted uranium. Zeolite has a negatively charged cage-like structure in which the radioactive particles become trapped. When the zeolite is excreted from the body through the normal channels of elimination, it takes with it the contaminants. It is available in the USA directly from Wairora; or simply get in touch with **Matt Twine**, who is based in the UK, but can handle all international and UK enquiries at this email address: **matt@zeoliteuk.co.uk**. His telephone number for the UK is: 01202 232493; International: (0044-1202-2324930).

Caution!
Zeolite is contraindicated for those taking medication containing heavy metals. If you have been diagnosed with

heavy metal toxicity, it is recommended that you seek the guidance of a suitably qualified practitioner before undertaking detoxification using zeolite, in order that you are guided through the process.

DID YOU KNOW?
Natural zeolite has been used in the clean-up of radioactive fall-out in Chernobyl and Three Mile Island.

Free Radicals

As we know, everything, whether living or non-living, is made up of tiny particles known as atoms. A group of atoms combined form a molecule. A good example is water which is a combination of hydrogen and oxygen atoms, expressed as H_2O.

Most atoms and molecules have an electrical charge which makes them stable. Conversely, the atoms or molecules known as free radicals are very unstable since they have an uneven electrical charge. This makes them highly reactive since they are constantly searching for other molecules with a positive charge in order to complete themselves. This is called oxidation.

Surprising as it may seem, the body constantly produces free radicals as a consequence of normal metabolism. Under normal circumstances this doesn't cause any problems. Sometimes, however, the body over-reacts and produces too many free radicals. Such over-production can be triggered by ultra-violet light, air pollution (e.g. cigarette smoke), illness, excessive exercise and radiation. Since free radicals have a tendency to oxidize they can damage cell membranes as well as DNA. This paves the way for disease to develop. Diseases such as hardening of the arteries, cancer, some forms of arthritis and high blood pressure, are linked with free radical damage. Free radicals are also associated with hastening of the ageing process.

Other significant sources of free radicals include pesticides, some food additives, pollution, hydrogenated fats and food fried in polyunsaturated oils (e.g. sunflower and safflower oils). This is because polyunsaturated oils have lots of double bonds (refer to Chapter 5) and free radicals love to latch on to these, the catalyst for the reaction being heat. For this reason it is advisable to limit consumption of fried foods and when you do fry, use the steam frying method. This involves cooking your food in a little water until just beginning to soften. You then add a little extra virgin olive oil or coconut oil and steam fry until the food is cooked. In this way you use less oil, without losing the taste benefits. Also, the oils are subjected to less heat compared to normal frying methods.

Nature's Defenders – the Antioxidants

Fortunately, as is often the case in nature, there are positive factors which can balance the negative factors. For instance, the body itself has a number of defense mechanisms which mop up excess free radicals. They include antioxidant enzymes and amino acids, cysteine and glutathione. Other anti-oxidant nutrients are derived from natural foods and include Vitamin C, beta carotene (the plant form of Vitamin A), Vitamin E found in wheat germ, avocados and seeds (such as sunflower and sesame) and the minerals zinc, iron, manganese, copper and selenium. Interestingly, nature ensures that foods such as oils found in nuts, seeds, whole grains and avocados, are protected from oxidation due to the presence of antioxidant nutrients such as Vitamin E.

Key antioxidants

The principle antioxidants include vitamins C, E, beta carotene, alpha lipoic acid, selenium, zinc and several natural compounds found in plants, otherwise known as phytochemicals; a good example would be carotenes found in highly colored foods such as sweet potatoes and carrots; also lycopene, found in foods like tomatoes.

If your child's diet is based largely upon natural foods, preferably organically grown; then he/she will automatically be provided with the best line of defense against many of the pollutants that represent a potential threat to their health. Having said this, the question is:

"Should we be happy to leave it at that, being content in the knowledge that we have done enough to protect our children?"

Many experts on nutrition firmly believe that we may not be getting enough protective nutrients, even from a natural diet. One such expert, Linus Pauling, who some considered to be one of the USA's greatest scientific minds, believed greatly in the healing power of Vitamin C. Always being the kind of person to practice what he preached, Pauling took several grams of Vitamin C every day of his life.

In some ways, Linus Pauling, by highlighting the value of supplementing one's diet with extra Vitamin C, helped to pave the way for research in to the value of other antioxidants.

Nowadays food scientists are becoming increasingly knowledgeable of the role that anti-oxidants play in the body, namely:

- As free radical scavengers, antioxidants help to mop up excess free radicals in the body.

- Detoxification – toxins such as drugs, pesticides, and food additives need to be rendered harmless to the body. Much of this detoxification is carried out by enzymes in the liver. Antioxidants are concentrated in the liver to aid in this process.

- Toxin Neutralizers – Many toxins, once inside the body, attempt to get incorporated into cells. Anti-oxidants help to directly neutralize these toxins, thus reducing their absorption. Vitamin C is known to be a very effective toxin neutralizer as well as having the capacity to latch onto harmful substances which can then be safely eliminated from the body. This is why Vitamin C is used to help people undergoing drug rehabilitation. It is also the reason why it's not a good idea to take large doses of Vitamin C prior to been administered anesthetics, as this may interfere with their effectiveness. This is why I would be careful to take this vitamin after dental treatment and not before.

How Antioxidant Levels of Natural Foods are Measured

As you would expect, the level of antioxidants present in different foods does vary, and thanks to the scientists at Tufts University in Boston, Massachusetts, it is now possible to measure the antioxidant capacities of a variety of foods.

This is a method called Oxygen Radical Absorbance Capacity (ORAC). In essence, this is a laboratory test that actually measures the ORAC capacity of different foods and natural substances. It is known as the ORAC scale, which is said to be one of the most accurate methods of measuring antioxidant capacity. What's really great about this type of measurement is that everyday natural foods are given an ORAC score; so we can see at a glance which foods have the greatest antioxidant capacity and subsequently include more of them in our diet and that of our children.

Early studies of the effects of adhering to a diet high in antioxidants have indicated several benefits including raised antioxidants levels in human blood; partial protection of long-term learning capacity and long-term memory in rats; and protection of rats' blood vessels from oxygen damage.

Not surprisingly, some scientists have postulated that the ability to determine ORAC measurements may arm us with the ability to manipulate our diets in order to prevent many diseases.

Here are some of the Best Antioxidant Foods with the greatest ORAC Scores:

FOODSERVING	SIZE	ANTIOXIDANT
Small red bean (dried)	½ cup	13727
Wild blueberry	1 cup	13427
Red kidney bean (dried)	½ cup	13269
Pinto bean	½ cup	11865
Cranberry	1 cup	8963
Artichoke hearts (cooked)	1 cup	7904
Blackberry	1 cup	7701
Dried prune	½ cup	7291
Raspberry	1 cup	6068
Strawberry	1 cup	6938
Apple - red Delicious	1 apple	6900
Apple - Granny Smith	1 apple	6381
Pecan	1 ounce	5095
Black bean (dried)	½ cup	4181
Plum	1 plum	4118
raw unprocessed cocoa	100g	28,000
Dark chocolate	100g	13,120
Milk chocolate	100g	none

These findings strongly reinforce the approach that we should be feeding our children a variety of fruits, vegetables, whole grains and pulses. By doing so, we will be ensuring that they receive a high level of protective antioxidants in a form that is recognised and easily absorbed by the body.

Also, research suggests that because they are naturally occurring substances, they work together much more effectively as a family; or to use the scientific expression, synergistically. This would certainly explain why, when these substances are tested individually, they do not always perform so effectively; for example, as is the case with beta carotene, and also vitamin E. In effect, the best way for your child to get antioxidants is through eating whole foods (preferably organically grown) in combination with a specially formulated antioxidant formula for children.

Important!

Pregnant women and those trying to concieve should avoid taking supplements that contain vitamin A due to increased risk of birth defects. If in doubt consult your family doctor.

Is Dark Chocolate Healthy?

Yes, it does appear to be true that dark chocolate is one of the best sources of antioxidants. In fact, raw unprocessed cocoa gets an ORAC rating of 28,000 per 100g, and dark chocolate gets a rating of 13,120 per 100g. Sadly, when the chocolate is processed to make milk chocolate, much of this value is lost. Candy bars and chocolate bars are not a health food. Nevertheless, I would say that a little chocolate, whether the dark variety or not, is not going to be too detrimental to your child. It is only when the consumption increases that we get problems, always remembering that cocao does contains stimulants which some children are more sensitive to than others.

Key Antioxidants for Children

The best way to ensure that your child is getting enough of the key antioxidants is to give them a broad spectrum vitamin and mineral supplement containing vitamins A,C,E, beta carotene, selenium and zinc. The formula may also contain cysteine and glutathione, and should also include other key vitamins and minerals, including vitamins D, B1, B2, B3, B5, B6, B12, folic acid, biotin and the minerals calcium, magnesium, iron, manganese and chromium. Furthermore, the mineral zeolite acts as an effective antioxidant (see 'Key Components of the Pollution Protection Programme' on page 189)).

What are the Best Vitamin Formulas for My Child?

Many nutritionists suggest that you should start supplementing your child's diet from the age of one year. It is best to choose a good chewable multivitamin and mineral formula that is not sweetened with sugar, except for a little fructose or sweetened with fruit extracts such as bilberry or grape. Very young children should have their chewable tablets ground into powder and added to their food. It is also advisable to add ground up seeds to your child's diet. This will add further calcium, magnesium plus essential fats.

The best companies do not add artificial anything to their formulas; so avoid those that contain substances such as artificial sweeteners (e.g. aspartame and saccharin).Most children's formulas give you a dosage according to the age of the child. This means that the older the child the more chewable tablets he/she needs to take on a daily basis.

Here is a list of reputable companies that produce children's supplements:

- Nature's Plus – This company produce a range of children's formulas designed for different age groups. They state that their chewables are 100% natural and contain no artificial colors, flavors, preservatives, yeast, wheat, corn, soy or milk. They also produce a wide range of other children's supplements. Website: www.naturesplus.com.

- Higher Nature – Their chewables are called Dinochews. As the name suggests, these are in the shape of dinosaurs. They contain natural flavors and claim that the nutrients in their formulas are at optimum levels. Higher Nature also produces a number of other children's supplements, including Essential Balance Junior – an excellent source of essential fatty acids, and a natural probiotic formula that provides helpful bacteria for the digestive system. Email:

customerservices@higher-nature.co.uk. Tel: 01435 884668.

- Biocare – This company offer a child's formula in capsule form that is suitable for children of 2 years and older. Their formula has been recommended by the Hyperactive Children's Support Group H.A.C.S.G. I would suggest that when it comes to very young children capsules should be broken open and sprinkled onto food in order to avoid the danger of choking. Email: sales@biocare. co.uk. Tel: 0121 4333727.

- Solgar USA; Solgar Inc. 500 Willow Tree Road, Leonia, NJ 07605 USA. Tel: 201-944-2311 Website: www.solgar.com/ Contacts.htm

- Another USA based company that might be worth checking out is Nature's Sunshine Products. Email: greatestherbs@gmail.com

- Blackmores; Australia, New Zealand and Eastern Asia; contact: 20 Jubilee Avenue, Warriewood NSW 2102, Australia. Tel: 61 2 9910 5000.

The Value of Exercise for Pollution Protection

Exercise has always been a big part of my life, and I have always tried to follow the 'use it or use it' philosophy. When we are young we instinctively run, skip, jump and enjoy the feeling of freedom and movement. In my own case, exercise was in the blood, right from the beginning. For some inexplicable reason, even as a toddler, I got into the habit of 'escaping' from the garden, and like a caged animal suddenly released from its restricted environment, I would run long distances; like some early version of Forest Gump. My parents would be in a panic, the police would be informed and relatives alerted.

One day, after unblocking the hole in the garden fence that had been repaired in a vain attempt to ensure my security, I escaped and started a marathon run that took me as far as a dual-carriageway over a mile away from my home. Fortunately for me my uncle Harold, out searching for me on his bicycle, halted my progress as I ran down the central reservation of the highway.

Thankfully, having now reached middle age, I have calmed down a bit. Of course, as we get older we tend to slow down and many of us learn to balance our lives so that exercise has a place in our daily routine, without being taken to excess.

Some people, children included, seem quite content to live sedentary lives, unaware of the dangers to their health that may be inherent in such a lifestyle.

Unfortunately, in today's society, there are more obese children than ever before. Generally speaking, children do not exercise as much as they did just a few decades ago. Couple this with a diet based upon junk foods, and in the longer term you have a recipe for ill health.

In terms of pollution protection, we have identified that a healthy body offers us a greater resistance against potential environmental threats. By introducing exercise into our children's lives, we are helping their ability to adapt to what has become an increasingly polluted world.

What Does Exercise Do for our Children?

The adage 'Movement is life, life is movement' makes a lot of sense. The fact is that the human body was built for movement, just as our brain was meant to think. When we don't exercise, our bodies begin to degenerate. This is obvious when we observe what happens to a leg that is immobilized in a plaster cast as a result of a bone fracture. After several weeks of entombment, when the cast is removed, we can easily notice a loss in muscle mass compared to the other leg.

Such muscle atrophy, as it's referred to, is perhaps not so apparent when it comes to your average 'couch potato'. Nevertheless, there will be deterioration in the condition of the musculature of the body and degeneration of the heart and lungs. Sadly, this isn't a scenario that just applies to us adults. Over the years, due to my involvement with teaching sports to children, I have observed from first hand the steady decline in fitness levels.

There are many reasons for this of course. Certainly, the diminishing role of PE and games in the school curriculum along with fewer safe areas for children to exercise hasn't helped. Nor have the hours that children devote to watching TV and playing on computer games. Add to this the fact that children are more likely to be driven from A to B instead of walking or cycling, and you are left with a generation of children lacking in fitness.

The most serious drawback associated with a lack of fitness in both adults and children, is the body's inability to extract oxygen from the atmosphere through breathing, and deliver it efficiently to all of the tissues, where it is used for energy. By engaging in regular sustained exercise over a period of time, we help to improve the body's capacity to transport and utilize oxygen.

In terms of building your child's resistance to potentially harmful toxins in the environment; regular exercise will result in the following benefits:

- The improved condition of the muscles in conjunction with good cardiovascular function results in more efficient detoxification of pollutants from the tissues.

- Improved circulation helps to ensure that a good supply of nutrients reach all parts of the body. Remember, many nutrients help to neutralize toxins.

- Moderate exercise helps to boost the immune system. A strong immune system = more resistance to pollution.

- Regular exercise will also usually result in better sleep patterns for those children who have trouble with sleeping. The greatest degree of detoxification occurs when we sleep.

- Exercise is a great antidote to stress. This is especially important during particularly stressful periods in your child's life; for example, when taking examinations at school. Prolonged stress can adversely affect the immune system.

How Much Exercise?

Generally speaking, any exercise which raises the heart rate for twenty minutes for a minimum of three times each week is good. Such activities as brisk walking, jogging, swimming, roller-skating, team sports and cycling are excellent for conditioning the muscles and strengthening the heart and lungs.

Resistance exercise, such as weight training, can be introduced from the age of about 16 years old. Some authorities on the subject warn against lifting heavy weights before this age in view of the fact that the skeleton is growing at a rapid rate for most children. If only I had been aware of this when I was a child, since I began competitive weightlifting when I was only 13 years old; a situation that would be discouraged these days.

Children can be brought up to be more conscious of exercise in daily activities; for instance, they can be encouraged to take the stairs instead of the elevator.

Recommended Exercises

Some of the best all-round exercises include brisk walking, swimming, skipping, jogging, cycling, circuit training, tennis, badminton, squash and athletics. Team sports such as basketball, netball, hockey, soccer, football and baseball are excellent for developing all-round strength and improved cardiovascular efficiency. Resistance training with weights can be introduced after the age of 16 years.

Important: If your child is overweight or has been used to living a sedentary lifestyle; it might be wise to arrange a general health check before they embark on an exercise regime.

Summary: the Key Components of the Pollution Protection Programme

- A natural diet comprising of fruits, vegetables, whole grains, nuts, seeds, pulses, fish and lean white meats.

- A suitable children's vitamin and mineral supplement.

- Use of freshly-made juices.

- Regular exercise.

- Taking steps to minimize exposure to pollutants; for example, use of a suitable water filter.

- By including natural food supplements such as chlorella and kelp.

- By using a reputable brand of zeolite, such as Waiora's NCD (natural cellular defense). Caution: do seek advice from Waiora regarding dosage instructions for children.

Conclusion

If there is one principle message that I wanted to convey in this book, it is this:

> When it comes to creating optimum health for your child, Nature really does know best.

In other words, as I hope it will be evident by now, our very genetic make up determines that we must adhere to certain natural laws in order to achieve and maintain, what is in effect, our birthright; namely that of freedom from disease and good health.

Of course, reaching an optimum level of wellness will be harder for some compared to others. This is usually determined by the constitution that we have inherited from our parents, in addition to the toxic load that we are subjected to both before and after birth.

With regard to the constitution, some people get what I refer to as an unlucky throw of the 'genetic dice'; conversely, others are much luckier and inherit the constitution of an ox. I suspect that the majority of folk are maybe somewhere in between.

However, whatever category your child may fall into, good health can only be achieved by sticking to the basic rules, which are encompassed within this book.

Finally, to all of those mums and dads out there who want the best for their priceless children, I hope the information in this book may make a small but significant contribution towards achieving your objective.

Useful Information

Nutrition

Chia seeds

A company called **Lifemax** has produced a very good chia seed product called MILA, which optimizes their nutritional value. In order to preserve the nutritional value of the seeds they use a patented machine that micro slices the seed with freeze cooled blades and the chia seeds are never heated in this process. They are based in the USA but are expanding into the UK and Europe. If you want to find out more or place an order for their product contact: **Kendra Epstein**. Her telephone number is: 314-368-5881. Website: www.kendraepstein.lifemax. net. Email: kendraepstein@mac.com.

Omega oil supplements

In the UK, Higher Nature offer a formula called Essential Balance Junior, which contains a good balance of Omega 3 and Omega 6 fats. This oil can also be purchased with butterscotch flavoring (all natural, I might add). Another good brand is Udo's Choice, which is available in several countries, including the USA, Australia, Europe and Canada. For further information see: www.udoerasmus.com

Supplement Companies

Herbal remedies

- A Vogel/Bioforce (UK) Ltd. Telephone: 01294 277344. Email: enquiries@bioforce.co.uk. International: info@bioforce.ch.

Health supplements

- Higher Nature. Telephone: 01435 883484. Email: info@ higher-nature.co.uk.

- Biocare. For UK sales, telephone: 0121 4333727. Email: sales@biocare.co.uk. Website: www.Biocare.co.uk.

- Solgar. Website: www.solgar.com. Email: international@ solgar.com.

- Nature's Sunshine Products, USA. Email: greatestherbs @gmail.com.

- For the chia seeds product Mila, contact: www.whati-flifemax.com. To order, contact: kendraepstein@mac.com.

USA residents may like to contact the Hippocrates Health Institute which is based in Florida. The address is: 1443 Palmdale Court, West palm Beach, FL 33411-3388. Telephone: 561-471-8876.

They produce a variety of natural supplements, including a natural source of B12, and it is worth asking their advice about a suitable supplement for children.

United Kingdom

Testing
Signs of Life: electro-dermal testing for:
    Food intolerances
    Environmental sensitivities (e.g. house-dust mite, printer's ink)
    Heavy metals
    Vitamin and mineral deficiencies
    Digestive function
    Parasites

For bookings call Signs of Life on: 07788710667 email: bio_cure@ hotmail.com.

YorkTest laboratories: test for food intolerances. They sell a home test kit for food and chemical allergies that require you to take a pinprick blood sample. Contact them to order a home test kit on freephone: 0800 074 6185. You can also view their website on: www.yorktest.com.

Parasite and stool analysis test

If you suspect that you or your child is suffering from a parasite infection, then you should consult a qualified Nutritional Practitioner. For a list of reputable practitioners contact BANT (British Association of Nutritional Therapists). Their telephone number is: 0870 606 1284; or view their website address: www. bant.org.uk. Or contact David Reavely on: 07788710667; email: bio_cure@ hotmail.com.

USA

Food intolerance testing

Contact: Cell Science Systems. Tel: (0800) US ALCAT (872-5228). Email: info@alcat.com.

If you want to look into Biomeridian Voll testing further you can email Biomeridian on: breceptionist@biomeridian.com. They are a USA based company and their address is: Biomeridian International, 2440 South 1070 West Suite A, Salt Lake City, Utah 84119.

Digestive problems

Based in the USA, The Great Smokies Diagnostic Laboratories carry out a Comprehensive Digestive Stool Analysis (CDSA). This identifies any underlying conditions that may be associated with conditions such as IBS (irritable bowel syndrome), indigestion, bloating etc. Tel: 800-522-4762.

Australia

Food intolerance testing. Contact: ImuPro. Tel: (Intl) +61 (0)2 9261 0688.

Recommended Books

The Optimum Nutrition Bible, Holford, P: Piatkus Books, 2004

Optimum Nutrition for your Child's Mind, Holford, P: Piatkus Books, 2006-11-30

Living Food – The Key to Health and Vitality, P. Holford: ION Press, 1996

Fats That Heal Fats That Kill, Dr. U. Erasmus: Alive Books, 1987/1994

Nutrition Counseling in the Treatment of Eating Disorders, M. Herrin: Brunner- Routledge, 2003

The Sprouter's Handbook, Cairney, E: Argyll Publishing; reprinted 2002

The Juicemaster's Ultimate Fast Food: Discover the Power of Raw Juice, Vale, J:HarperCollins, 2003

The Jan de Vries Guide to Health and Vitality; de Vries, J: Trafalgar Square, 2006

The Chemical Maze Shopping Companion, Statham, B. Summersdale Publishers Ltd, 2006

The Big Fat Mystery – how hidden food intolerances could be sabotaging your attempts to lose weight; Reavely, D. Metro Books, 2008

The Complete Idiot's Guide to Vegan Eating for Kids, Villamagna, Dana & Andre, Penguin, 2010

Dr Jensen's Juicing Therapy, Dr Jensen, B, McGrawHill, 2000

Deadly Harvest, The Intimate Relationship Between Our Health And Our Food, Bond, G, SquareOne Publishers, 2007

Brain Building Nutrition, How Dietary Fats and Oils Affect Mental, Physical and Emotional Intelligence, Schmidt, M, A, Frog Books, Ltd

Natural Cosmetics Companies

- Dr. Hauschka Skin Care. For enquiries contact: enquiries@ drhauschka.co.uk. Telephone UK: 01386 791022.

- Green People – organic skincare. Website: www.green-people. co.uk.

- Jurlique: USA: customercare@jurlique.com. Address: Jurlique Skin Care, One Bridge Street, Suite 42, Irvington, NY 10533, United States. Jurlique: UK: Holly House, 300-302 Chiswick High Road, London W4 1NP. Website: www.jurlique.co.uk. Jurlique: Australia: Jurlique, 52-54 Oborn Road, Mount Barker, SA 5251. Email: pr@jurlique. com.

- Weleda Skin Care Products: www.weleda.com.

- Higher Nature – see under Health Supplements, above.

Useful Organizations

- Mount Sinai Environmental Health Center (CEHC) based in the USA. They conduct research to discover the environmental causes of disease in children – for example, asthma, learning disabilities, autism, obesity and child cancer. They convey their research findings to pediatricians, policy makers, child carers and parents. Tel: 212-824-7125. Email: info@cehcenter.org.

- The Environmental Working Group. For more information on food pesticide levels contact them at: Headquarters: 1436 U Street. NW, Suite 100 / Washington, DC 20009 / (202) 667-6982. Website: www.ewg.org.

Natural Health Practitioner Organizations

- The British Naturopathic Association – for list of reputable Naturopaths in your locality. Telephone: 0870 745 6984.

- American Naturopathic Medical Association: ANMA, P.O. Box 96273, Las Vegas, Nevada 89193. Telephone: (702) 897-7053.

- Australian Naturopathic Practitioners Association: ANPA, Suite 36/123 Cambewell Road, East Hawthorn, Victoria 3123, Australia. Telephone: + 613 9811 9990. Email: admin@anpa.asn.au.

- The British Association of Nutritional Therapists (BANT) – for list of registered practitioners in your area. Email: the administrator@bant.org.uk. Telephone: 08706 0611284.

- Canada: World Organization of Natural Medicine www.wonmfoundation.org

- Czech: Kneipp Hydrotherapy and Naturopathic Therapy www.kneipp.ch

- Denmark: Danish Nature-cure Federation www.danskheilpraktikerforening.dk

- European Federation for Naturopathy www.effn.org

- French Federation of Naturopathy www.fenahman.org

- Professional Association of German Naturopaths www.heilpraktiker.org

- Union of German Naturopaths
  www.heilpraktiker-vdh.de/

- Italian Federation for Naturopathy
  www.fenai.it

- New Zealand Society of Naturopaths
  www.naturopath.org.nz/index.html

- Portuguese Association of Naturopathy
  www.fenaman.net

- Switzerland: Amalgamated Natural Physicians
  www.naturaerzte.ch

- Association of Swiss Naturopaths and Therapists
  www.naturopati.ch/

- Switzerland: Kneipp Hydrotherapy and Naturopathic
  Therapy
  www.kneipp.ch/

- Spanish Federation of Professional Naturopaths
  www.fenaco.net/inicio.htm

- Netherlands: European Action for Freedom of Therapy
  and the Right to Health
  www.eghealth.org

Radiation, Electricity Pylons and Telephone Masts

If you have concerns about working or living in close proximity
to a base station or mast, or other concerns relating to EMF's or
microwave radiation exposure; there are organizations that you
can contact for advice.

If you are a resident of the USA, then contact

The **Environmental Protection Agency**
Ariel Rios Building
1200 Pennsylvania Avenue, N.W.
Washington DC 20460
(202) 272-0167
TTY (speech and hearing impaired) (202) 272-0165

Those readers resident in the UK can seek information by contacting the organization **Powerwatch**

2 Tower Road
Sutton
Ely
Cambridgeshire CB6 2QA
www.powerwatch.org.uk